DIET AND DIABETES

By the same author :

- जीवन मधुमेह के संग
- हृदय रोग और आप: रोग, उपचार एवं सावधानियाँ
- डायबिटीज प्रश्नोत्तरी
- Diet And Diabetes
- You And Your Diabetes
- Diabetes Quiz Book

About the Author

Dr. Ashok K. Jhingan, (*b.* 1949) M.B.B.S., M.D. Medicine has worked as Senior Consultant in Medicine Deptt. in Jaipur Golden Hospital and National Heart Institute and is a visiting Consultant in Sir Ganga Ram Hospital, Delhi. At present he is also a consultant Diabetologist with BHEL.

Author started working in the field of Diabetes since 1983 and has been organised Diabetes Detection and Education Camps in and around Delhi.

Author is a firm believer of the fact that Diabetics who know more about diabetes can live longer.

Author has written six books on diabetes and heart problems (in Hindi and English). These books have been appreciated by masses and this is evident from the fact that their new editions had to be brought out.

Delhi Diabetes Research Centre (DDRC) is a registered society and was established by group of doctors from India and abroad along with diabetes Educators and Nutrition Experts. Its sole aim is to help and educate Diabetics by arranging regular seminars and conferences, so that they can lead normal life with diabetes. So far we have organised 130 such camps in and around Delhi. Every year we organize 3 day Diabetes Health Melas which is being attended by thousands of people. These melas have created diabetes awareness in masses.

2nd Revised & Enlarged Edition

DIET AND DIABETES

Dr. Ashok K. Jhingan
M.B.B.S., M.D. (Medicine), FIAMS
Chairman
Delhi Diabetes Research Centre (DDRC)

CONCEPT PUBLISHING COMPANY PVT. LTD.,
NEW DELHI-110059

ISBN-13 : 978-81-8069-878-1

2nd Revised & Enlarged Edition 2012

Published and Printed by

Concept
Since 1974

Concept Publishing Company Pvt. Ltd.
A/15-16, Commercial Block, Mohan Garden
New Delhi-110059 (India)
T: 25351460, 25351794, *F*: 091-11-25357109
E: publishing@conceptpub.com, W: www.conceptpub.com
Editorial Office: H-13, Bali Nagar, New Delhi-110 015, India.

Cataloging in Publication Data--*Courtesy:* D.K. Agencies (P) Ltd. <docinfo@dkagencies.com>

Jhiṅgana, E. Ke. (Aśoka Ke.), 1949-
Diet and diabetes / Ashok K. Jhingan. — 2nd rev. & enl. ed.
p. cm.
ISBN 9788180698781

1. Diabetes—Nutritional aspects. 2. Diabetes—Popular works. 3. Diet in disease. I. Jhingan, author. II. Title.

DDC 616.462 23

This book is dedicated with deepest love and affection to my parents. Their love, wisdom and strength have always been a source of inspiration for me.

Preface

We are witnessing a global epidemic of diabetes and obesity, and, in their wake, of cardiovascular and renal disease. Prevention and treatment will require an in-depth understanding of therapeutic options. It is therefore timely and appropriate that this book has been dedicated to the topic of Nutrition and Plate Method. Diet plays important role when Diabetic develops Renal disease or heart problem.

In the first part I have tried to give detail information about carb counting, calories, carbohydrates, fats and protein and disadvantage about over cooking. Detailed information about use of oil and artificial sweeteners have also been shared in this edition. I am thankful to Dr. Ram Mohan M.D. for sharing latest information about calorie fat and carbohydrates counting.

26 November, 2011 **Dr. Ashok K. Jhingan**

Contents

Diabetes

Diabetes Mellitus is a chronic metabolic disorder with strong hereditary basis, associated with high glucose and usually passage of sugar in urine.

There is no disease, which provokes greater thought on diet than diabetes. Many diabetics unable to follow strict diet regimen for the rest of their lives, try pills, herbs, and infusions recommended by friends who claim to have tried them and become symptom free without diet control. These items are claimed to be so effective that even follow up examination for sugar are declared unnecessary. The euphoria continues till suddenly a complication of Diabetes like Heart Disease, Coma or stroke occurs.

Diabetes is no longer a dreaded disease; a well-managed diabetic has a good life expectancy. Diet is a sheet anchor of treatment in obese Type II diabetics, and a useful supplement to insulin therapy in younger ones.

Basic Factors in Planning a Diet

1. Lifestyle: work schedule and exercise routine.
2. Medication: insulin or oral medication.
3. Weight goal: need to gain weight, loose weight or maintain weight.
4. Medical conditions any associated medical problem or not.
5. Food preferences: veg or non-veg.

What to Eat

Since your body is having trouble getting energy from the food you eat, it is important to know the nutritional values of food, so that a nutritious healthy, energy giving diet can be devised which not only gives proper nutrition but also controls your blood sugar levels with a benefit of being able to eat your favourite food.

Basic Dietary Guidelines

1. Eat variety of foods.
2. Maintain desirable weight.
3. Avoid extra fat, particularly saturated fats and cholesterol rich food.
4. Eat foods with adequate fibres.
5. If you take insulin, coordinate your food intake with the action of insulin.
6. Avoid too much salt as in processed and fast foods.
7. Avoid eating sugar and starchy food.

Reshaping Eating Behaviours

- Eating is a behaviour that is largely controlled by people with whom we live or socialize, place where we live and our emotions. Become aware of those situations that commonly lead to extra food being eaten.
- We may also be unaware of 'bad' eating habits that can lead to excess calorie intake; e.g. eating quickly, large mouthfuls, eating when tense or bored, finishing a large serving of food when not hungry.

Practice saying 'NO' politely but assertively.

Tips to help uncover and correct 'BAD' eating habits:

- **Don't eat while engaged in other activities;** for example watching TV, reading and nibbling at snacks while chit-chatting. Eat only at the dining table, not near the fridge.
- **Don't eat quickly.** Chewing slowly allows time to register a feeling of fullness. Cut food into smaller pieces. Don't load your fork until the previous mouthful is finished.
- **Don't purchase high calorie foods.** Shop from a set list to prevent impulse buying. Avoid shopping with children.
- **Buy snack foods** in the smallest package. The larger the serving size or package, the more you are likely to eat or drink.
- **Plan meals in advance. Stick to a set menu.**

> Do you use food as an emotional crutch? If so, professional counselling may be helpful.

1. **Plan a strategy to avoid uncontrolled eating** and drinking at social events, or when your emotions urge you to binge.
   Rehearse repeatedly in your mind exactly what you will do in such situations. Remind yourself several times each day that you are in charge of your actions and that you can be strong-willed. Seek counseling or coaching on various strategies.
2. **Distract yourself** when you feel the urge to snack impulsively. Engage in some activity that will distract you from thinking about food. Examples: go for a walk, brush your teeth, phone a friend.
   If you eat out of boredom, find some new hobby or interest that gets you out of the house. Even enroll in an adult education class.
3. **Recording your eating and exercise habits** jolts you into realizing just what you do eat and drink each day; and also whether you exercise sufficiently.

(i) **Helps you identify problem foods** and drinks with excessive calories and fat.

(ii) **Helps identify moods,** situations and events that lead to excessive eating of unwanted calories. You can then plan to overcome or avoid them.

(iii) **Prevents 'calorie amnesia',** the forgetfulness that leads to rebound weight gain after successful weight loss. Recording puts you back on the right tract.

(iv) **Helps you develop greater self-discipline.** You will think twice about overindulging if you have to record it—especially if someone checks your journal regularly. It certainly keeps you honest!

(v) **Motivates you** to carefully plan your meals and to exercise each day.

(vi) **Serves as a check system** for your doctor, dietician or counselor to assess your progress and make recommendations.

Diabetes Guide

What is Diabetes?

Diabetes occurs when the body has difficulty processing glucose (sugar) in the blood.

- **After digestion,** sugar and starches are changed into **glucose**—the simplest form of sugar, vital for body energy and growth.
- Insulin is the hormone which acts like a key that opens the door to body cells and allows glucose to enter.
- **Without enough insulin,** glucose builds up in the blood and passes into the urine. High blood glucose levels lead to frequent urination, extreme thirst, and tiredness.
- **Untreated diabetes increases the risk of damage to nerves and blood vessels.** This, in turn, increases the risk of heart disease, stroke, blindness, kidney damage, foot ulcers and gangrene, impotence and other complications.

Symptoms of Diabetes

- Frequent urination
- Extreme thirst
- Unusual hunger
- Rapid weight loss
- Extreme fatigue
- Blurred vision
- Skin infections that are slow to heal
- Tingling/numbness in feet

Note : Diabetes can occasionally be present even without any symptoms.

Type 1 Diabetes

- Occurs in 10% of diabetes cases
- Usually in children and young adults
- Pancreas produces little or no insulin. Daily insulin injections (or use of an insulin pump) are necessary, as well as:
  - matching pre-meal insulin to the amount of carbohydrate eaten
  - weight control and regular physical activity

> Insulin acts like a key. It opens the door to body cells and allows glucose to enter.
> People with type 1 diabetes and some with type 2 have too few or no keys and require insulin injections.
> Others (primarily type 2) make enough insulin but the body doesn't use it as well as it should—particularly if obese and inactive patients.

Type 2 Diabetes

- Occurs in 90% of diabetes cases
- Occurs mainly in adults—particularly in overweight and inactive persons
- Insulin is produced but body cells resist its action and glucose cannot enter cells
- Usually treated with meal planning and physical activity. Requires medication (pills or insulin) if blood sugar very high.

Gestational Diabetes

- Occurs in some women during pregnancy. It usually disappears after the baby's birth.
- Women who have had gestational diabetes still have a high risk of developing type 2 diabetes within 5 to 10 years.
- Requires weight control, a healthy lifestyle and regular medical checks.

Are you At Risk for Diabetes?

Pre-Diabetes—An Early Warning!

Pre-diabetes means that your blood glucose levels are higher than normal, but not high enough to be called diabetes.

If you have pre-diabetes, you have a higher risk for getting diabetes later on.

The good news is that you can start taking steps to prevent diabetes by making healthy lifestyle changes—such as losing weight if overweight, and being more physically active.

What's Your Risk?

Find out if you're at risk for diabetes by answering the following questions:

- ❑ I have been told I have pre-diabetes
- ❑ I have a family history of diabetes
- ❑ I am Asian, African, American, Latino American, Asian American, Native American
- ❑ I have had gestational diabetes (diabetes during pregnancy)
- ❑ I am over age 45
- ❑ I am overweight
- ❑ I get little or no physical activity
- ❑ My waist is larger than: 80 cms (for a woman) or 90 cms (for a man)
- ❑ My blood pressue is higher than 130/85 mm of Hg
- ❑ My HDL (good cholesterol) is too low
- ❑ My triglycerides (blood fats) are too high

Check Your Result

- If you've put a check mark in two or more of the boxes, you may be more likely to develop type 2 diabetes.
- Talk with your healthcare provider to see if you should have blood test for diabetes.

Blood Glucose Classfication of Diabetes

Normal	:	Below 100 mg/dl*
Pre-Diabetes	:	100-125 mg/dl*
Diabetes	:	Over 125 mg/dl*

(* Fasting Blood Glucose)

Know Your BGL (Blood Glucose Level): Everyone over the age of 45 should have a blood glucose test every three years.

Importance of Weight Control

- **Type 2 diabetes** is more common in people who are overweight.
- **Being overweight** means that your insulin doesn't work as well to control blood glucose levels.
- **Losing just 10 to 20 pounds** can help you better manage your diabetes and lower your risk for heart disease.

Keys to weight control include:

- Following a healthy eating plan
- Controlling food portions
- Being physically active most days of the week
- Keeping food records
- Setting realistic goals
- **Work with a registered dietitian** who can help you reach a weight that's ideal for you.

Keep Moving!

Everyday, do at least 30 minutes of moderate intensity exercise. (even in 5-minute sets) It's the key to improving insulin action. Add muscle strength training 3-4 times a week to double the benefits.

Managing Diabetes

Don't battle diabetes alone. Establish a partnership with your doctor, dietitian, certified diabetes educator, and pharmacist.

Hints to keep blood glucose within safe limits:

- **Control your food intake.** Know what and when you will eat. Consult a dietitian for expert advice.
- **Exercise regularly.** It assists weight control and can improve sensitivity of body cells to insulin. Plan physical activity into your daily routine.
- **Monitor your blood glucose** at home and work with a blood glucose meter. It will help you become familiar with your blood glucose patterns, and the effects of food, activity and medication.
- **Take insulin or oral medication as prescribed.** If on insulin, know what action to take if hypoglycemia (low blood glucose) occurs. Also educate your family and friends.

Be Heart Smart—Know Your ABC's

If you have diabetes, you are at a higher risk for heart attack and stroke than someone without diabetes. But you can fight back!

Be smart about your heart!

Take control of the ABC's of diabetes and live along and healthy life. Talk to your healthcare provider about your ABC targets.

A is of A1C

The A1C (A-one-C) test—short for hemoglobin A1C. It reflects your average blood glucose (sugar) over the last 3 months.

Suggested target: Below 7%

B is for Blood Pressure

High blood pressure makes your heart work too hard. **Suggested Target: Below 120/80**

C is for Cholesterol

Bad cholesterol, or LDL, can build up and clog your artieries. **Suggested Target: Below 100.**

Guidelines for choosing a healthy diet apply equally to people with or without diabetes. Eating a wide variety of foods that are mainly low in fat, low in refined sugars, and high in fiber, is recommended.

However, actual food quantities, as well as when you eat, will also influence control of blood glucose. Your dietitian will individualize a meal plan to suit your food preferences, lifestyle and medical status.

Eat a well-balanced diet with foods high in fiber and low in saturated fat.

Here are a few tips:

- **Maintain a healthy weight.** If overweight, even a modest weight loss plus daily physical activity can help manage blood glucose in type 2 diabetes.
- **Don't skip meals.** If you take insulin or an oral hypoglycemic agent, regular meals are important.

  If on insulin, eat meals at the same time each day. Eat a similar amount of food at each meal. Eating about the same amount of carbohydrate over the day will make best use of insulin and prevent wide variations in blood glucose levels.
- **Know which foods contain carbohydrate;** and learn how to check the *Nutrition Facts Label* on foods. Check the serving size, total fat and total carbohydrate—not just the sugar content. All carbohydrate breaks down to sugars after digestion.
- **Choose wholegrain breads, cereals and pasta.** Eat fresh fruits, vegetables and legumes. These foods contain more fiber and slow the release of glucose into your blood after a meal.
- **Limit foods high in saturated fats, trans fats and cholesterol.** Enjoy fish, soy foods, and other foods rich in omega-3 fats.
- **Limit sugars and foods high in added sugar** particularly if overweight. Small amounts of sugar as part of a meal may occasionally be okay. Check with your dietitian.

Alcohol Tips

- If you drink alcohol, have only moderate amounts:
  Men—1-2 drinks/day
  Women—1 drink/day
  For some people, safe drinking will mean no alcoholic drinks at all.
- **Drink along with your food**—especially if you use insulin or diabetes pills.
- **Do not omit any carb food** in exchange for an alcoholic drink. However, non-alcoholic beers (12 fl oz) count as one carb·exchange.
- **Alcohol increases the risk of hypoglycemia** (low blood sugar) and drug interactions if you take insulin and certain types of diabetes pills.
- **Check with your doctor and dietitian.**

The Plate Method—An Easy Way to Eat Healthfully

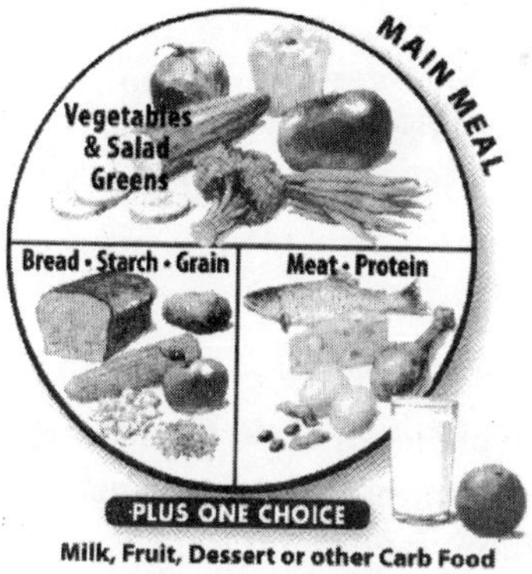

The plate method is a helpful tool to guide your food choices until you see a dietitian for your own meal plan.

For a healthy meal:

- Fill half of your plate with non-starchy vegetables (broccoli, green beans, carrots).
- Fill a quarter of your plate with carbhohydrate (wholegrain bread, pasta, potato, brown rice).

- Fill the other quarter of your plate with 3-4 ounces of lean meat, poultry, or fish.
- Add a small piece of fruit or 8 ounces of skim/low-fat milk or yogurt.

How Much Carbohydrate Should You Eat?

A dietitian can best determine how much carbohydrate you need at each of your meals, based on your lifestyle, food preferences, and overall diabetes control.

Until you see a dietitian, aim to keep the amount of carbohydrate you eat the same at each of your meals.

Carb Choices Meal Plan One Carb Choice = 15 Grams of Carb

The amount in: 1 slice Bread or ¾ cup Cereal (unsweetened) or 1 small Potato or 1 small fruit

Breakfast

- Eat 2-3 carb choices (30-45 grams)
- Include a low-fat protein source such as egg whites or skim milk.

Lunch and Dinner

- Eat 3-4 carb choices (45-60 grams carb)
- Include fruit and non-starchy vegetables. Choose small portions of low-fat protein foods.

Snacks

If needed, eat 1-2 carb choices (15-30 grams carb).

Note: Above plan is for adults. Carbohydrate amounts will vary with physical activity level.

Carb Type Affects Blood Glucose

The various forms of carbohydrate affect blood glucose levels in different ways. It is difficult to predict the effect of particular foods, sugars, or meals, simply by their carbohydrate content.

Thus the same amount of carbohydrate from different foods may affect blood sugar levels very differently. Many factors affect the rate of digestion and absorption such as:

- the type of sugar, starch, and fiber
- the degree of processing and cooking (which increases digestion rate)
- the amount of protein and fat (which slow stomach emptying and digestion).

Glycemic Index (GI)

The GI is a method of ranking carbohydrate foods on a scale (0-100) according to how they affect blood glucose levels. (See next column).

The higher the GI value, the greater the food's ability to rapidly raise blood glucose levels, and the more insulin needed by the body.

Eating low-GI foods may lead to better control of blood glucose and insulin levels (which in turn lowers the risk of damage to blood vessels and nerves). The slower digestion of low-GI foods may also help to delay hunger pangs and benefit weight control.

Cautionary Notes on GI

Choosing low-GI foods is not a license to eat unlimited amounts. Calorie restriction and portion control for weight control is of prime importance.

Also remember, Low-GI foods are carbohydrate foods and must still be counted as part of any dietetic carbohydrate plan.

GI is not meant to be used by itself without regard to portion size, and other dietary recommendations for healthy eating. Foods are not good or bad on the basis of their glycemic index (GI).

While GI may be a helpful tool for some people with diabetes, what is most important is to control the total amount of carbohydrate that you eat.

Lower-Glycemic Foods

Slower-Acting Carbohydrates: These foods are more slowly digested and absorbed. They help maintain more even blood glucose levels, as long as excessive amounts are not eaten. Use these foods regularly but still limit portion size for weight control.

Examples:

- Dried beans, peas, lentils
- Nuts and seeds
- Wholegrain breads
- Bran cereals, oats
- Sweet Corn, barley, buckwheat
- Wholegrain pasta, basmati rice
- Fresh fruit: apples, avacados, bananas (firm), cherries, grapefruit, olives, oranges, peaches, pears, plums. Fresh juices.
- Vegetables: broccoli, yam, sweet potatoes, salad greens
- Milk, yogurt, soy-drinks
- Dark chocolate

Higher-Glycemic Foods

Quicker-Acting Carbohydrates: These foods more rapidly raise blood glucose levels. Eat only in moderation.

- White bread, rice cakes, bagels, croissants, doughnuts
- Low-fiber cereals: Cornflakes, Rice Krispies.
- White potatoes, white rice
- Watermelon, ripe bananas, cantaloupe, pineapple
- Soda, sugar-sweetened sports and energy drinks
- Sugar, candy, popcorn (plain)
- Icecream (low-fat), frozen yogurt.

> High-GI fruits and potatoes are still healthy choices when eaten in moderate amounts.

What is Diabetes?

We need energy to live. Our body gets energy from the food we eat. People who have diabetes cannot utilize food in a proper way to give them energy.

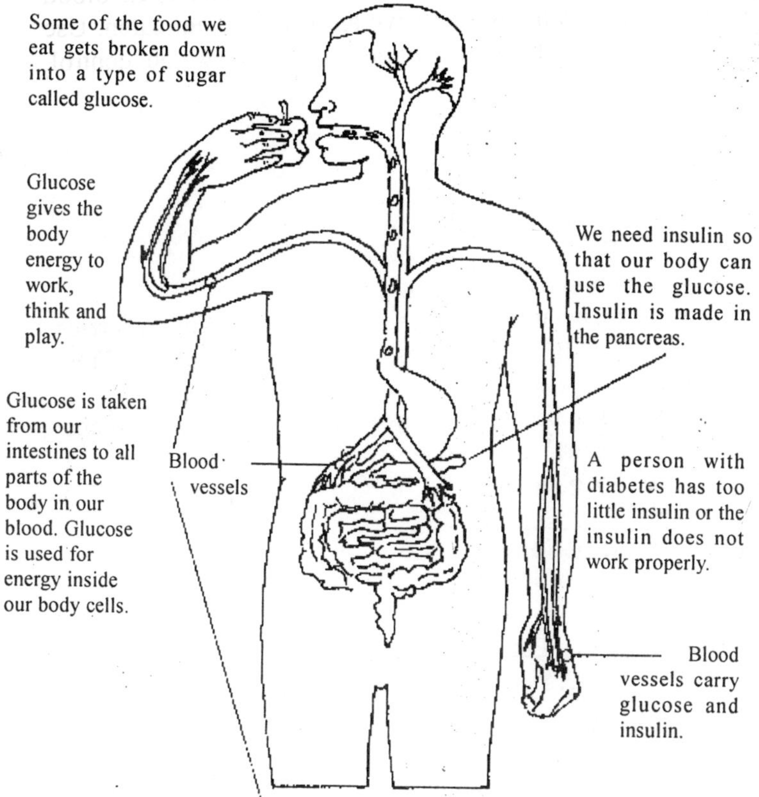

How insulin works?

Insulin is like a key that opens the door to allow glucose from the blood into the body cells.

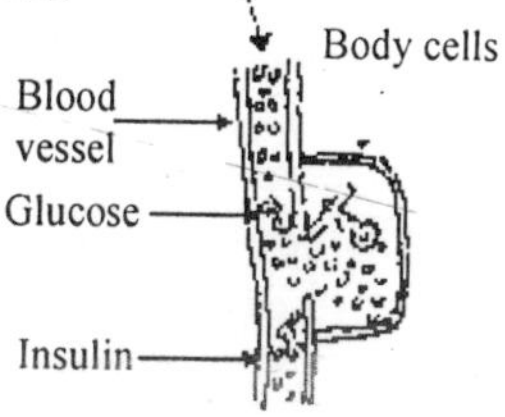

If there is not enough insulin the glucose stays in the blood. This means that the body cells get no energy.

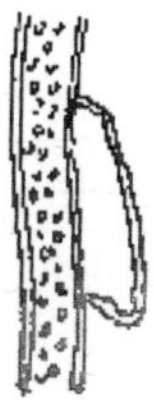

Signs of Diabetes

Here are some of the health problems that can be caused by diabetes. If you have any of these problems go to your doctor and ask to be tested for diabetes.

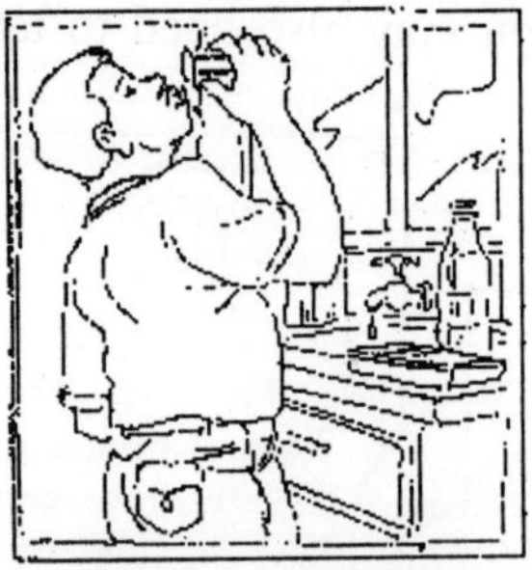

• Feeling very, very thirsty

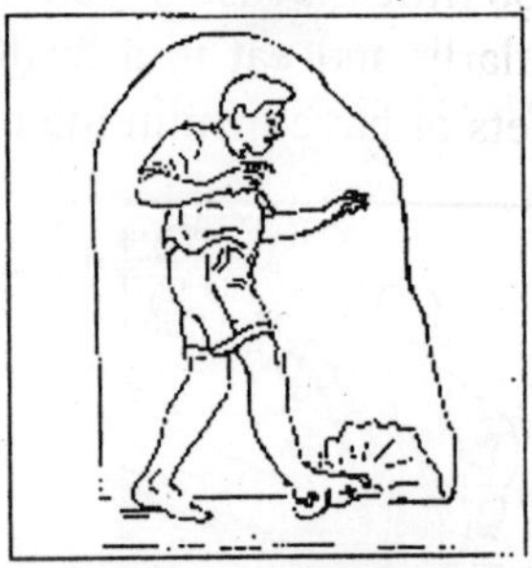

• Sores and boils that do not heal

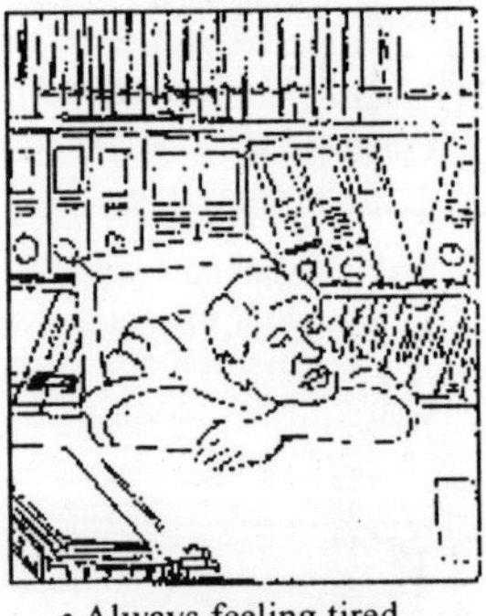

• Always feeling tired
• Not seeing well
• Losing weight even though you eat well
• Itching at private parts
• Impotence

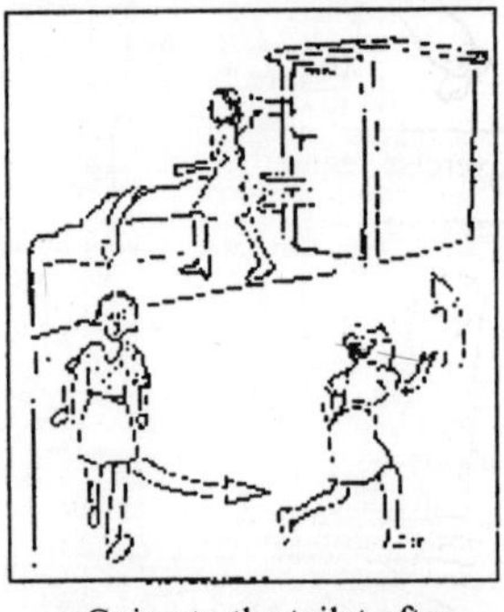

• Going to the toilet often

Some people with Diabetes have no symptoms
If diabetes is not treated it can lead to more serious problems like:

• blindness
• kidney failure
• heart attacks and strokes
• amputation of legs and feet

If you know what to do and get the right treatment these problems can be avoided!

Some people are more likely to get diabetes than others. Get your Blood Sugar tested if you are over 40, overweight and do not exercise. If you have family members with diabetes you should have a diabetes test every year.

Managing Diabetes

If you have diabetes you have to make sure that the level of glucose in your blood is within normal limits and not too much or too little glucose in your blood. To do this you need to exercise regularly and eat in a healthy way. You may also need to take tablets or have insulin injections.

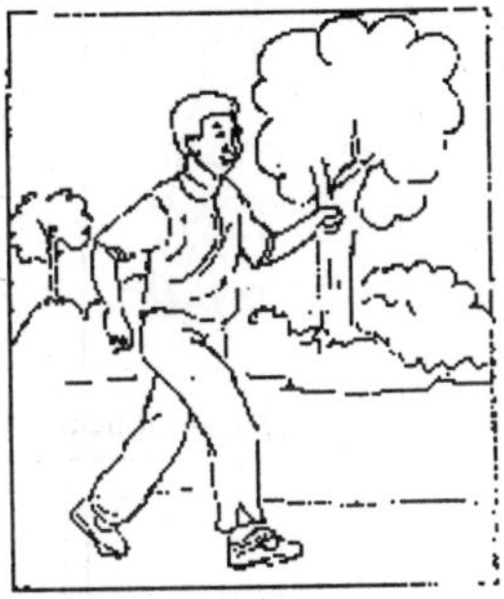

• Exercise regularly

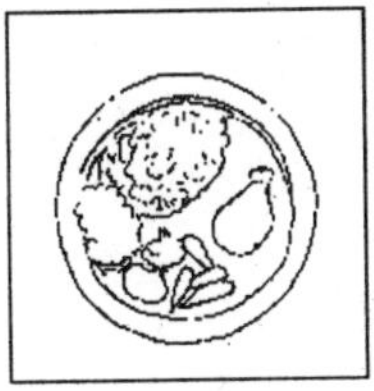

• Eat small, regular healthy meals

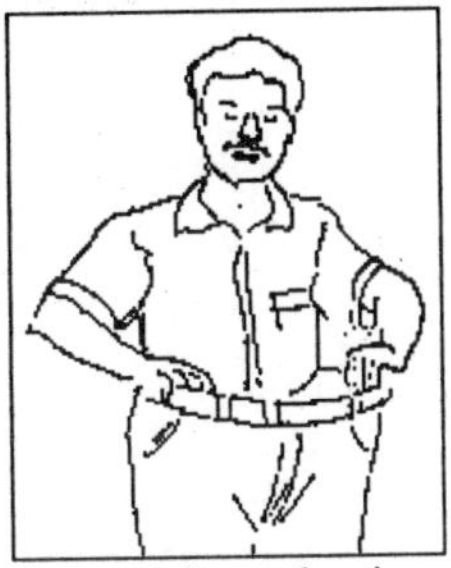

• Exercising and eating balanced diet will help you to lose weight

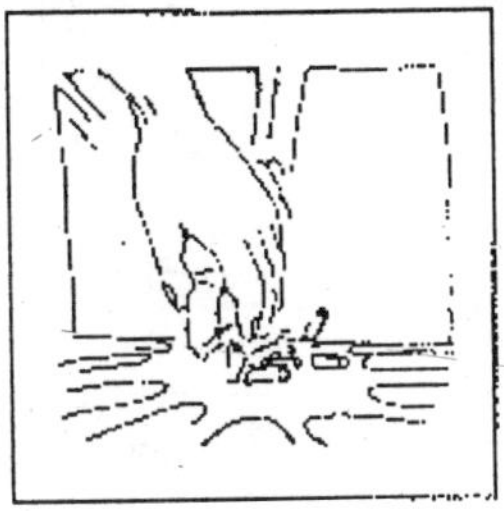

• Don't smoke

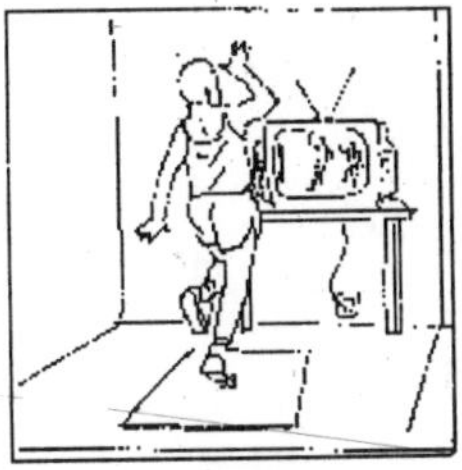

• Exercise helps

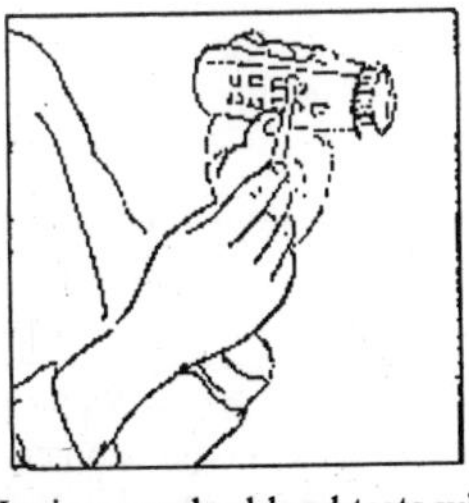

• Having regular blood tests will help to show if you are managing your diabetes correctly

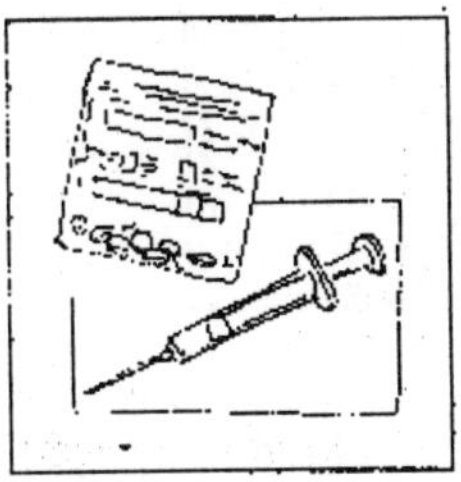

• Take tablets or insulin injections if your doctor recommends them

Looking after Yourself

If you have diabetes your body can easily get infections. Small injuries can develop into serious problems if they are not noticed and taken care of at an early stage.

Looking after Your Feet

Diabetes can reduce the flow of blood to your feet and make them cold. It can also cause loss of feeling in your feet.

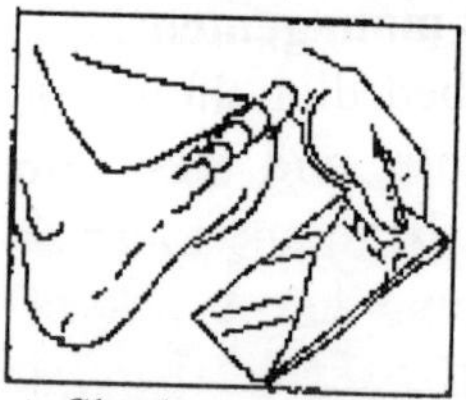

• Check your feet carefully everyday (go to the clinic if you have sores that won't heal)

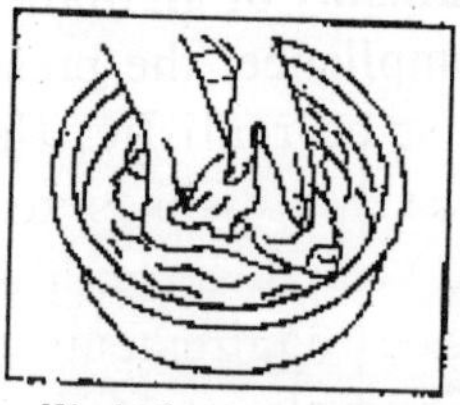

• Wash feet everyday in warm (not hot) water.

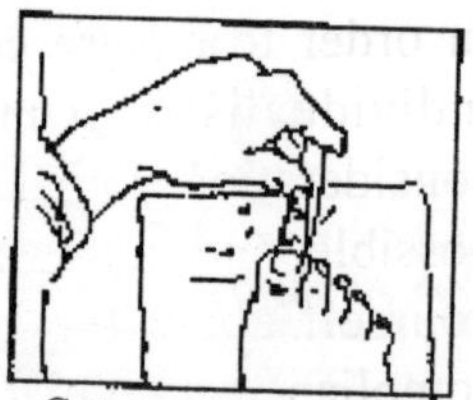

• Cut toe nails straight across

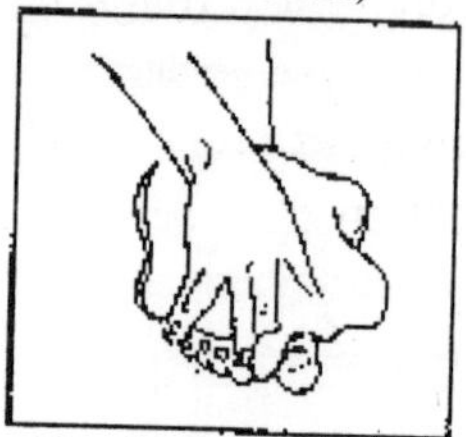

• Dry feet well especially between toes

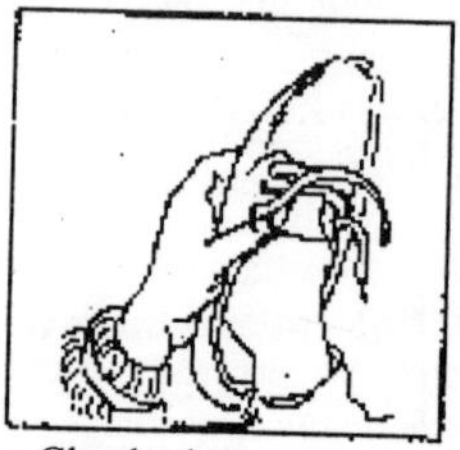

• Check shoes everyday for nails and stones

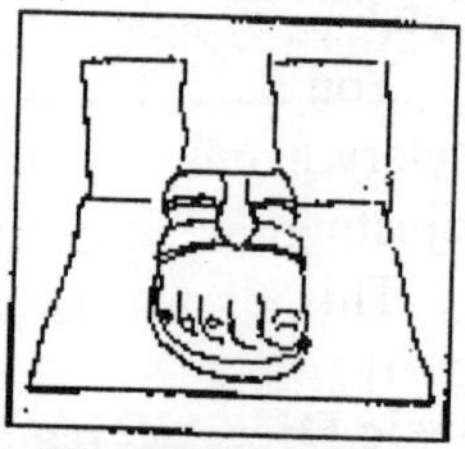

• Wear comfortable, well-fitting shoes or sandals

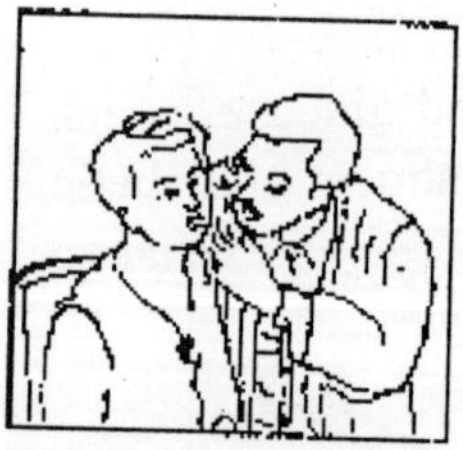

Looking after your eyes

High blood sugar may affect your eyesight. If you notice any changes in your eyesight go to see a doctor at the clinic. Have your eyes tested once a year, even if your vision has not changed

Looking after your mouth

Brush your teeth at least twice a day. Visit your dentist regularly and tell him that you have diabetes.

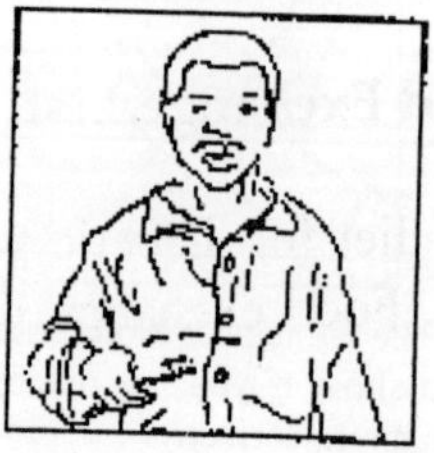

Diet in Diabetes

Diet Prescription

Diet should be the mainstay of all diabetes management! In order to ensure compliance, the prescribed diet should be individualised. It must be realistic, flexible, and take into consideration your likes and dislikes, to as large an extent as possible, and must suit your lifestyle. It is important to educate yourself about the basic requirements of the diet and judge compliance at regular intervals.

Interestingly, our traditional Indian diets with slight modifications are close to what is now considered ideal diabetic diets!

You do not have to make any major changes to your usual dietary habits with the exception of avoiding simple sugars and adjusting the fat intake.

This allows increasing compliance with the diet advised.

Basic Diet Advice

Avoid simple carbohydrates like sugar, sweets, jaggery, honey, etc. as they tend to cause a sharp rise in blood glucose levels. Dietary measures are an essential part of the treatment of diabetic patients. If a fixed daily intake is to be achieved an exchange system is necessary.

Food Exchange List

The diet for diabetic patient is prescribed in terms of exchange lists. Food exchange lists are groups of measured foods of the same calorific value and similiar protein, fat or carbohydrates and can be substituted one for another in a meal plan. All foods of exchange make a specific contribution to a good diet.

The food exchange lists help the paitent

(a) to restrict the food intake according to the insulin prescription so that both hyperglycemia and hypoglycemia can be prevented.
(b) to have variety in the diet so that he/she can adhere to it always.
(c) and easy learning of the principles of diet.

By following the food exchange list, diabetics can also maintain body weight.

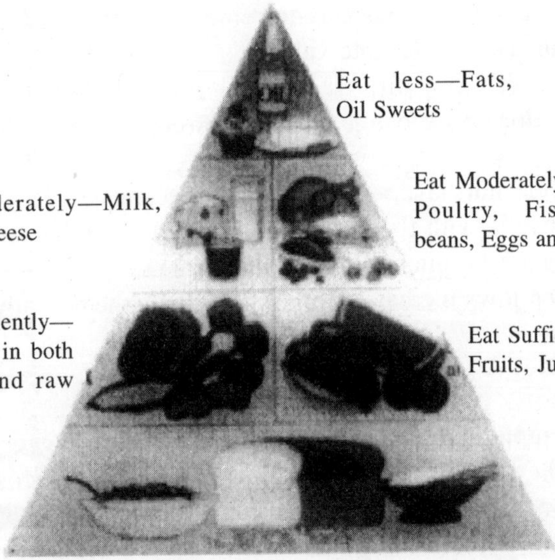
Eat less—Fats, Oil Sweets
Eat Moderately—Milk, Curd, Cheese
Eat Moderately—Meat, Poultry, Fish, Dry beans, Eggs and Nuts
Eat sufficiently—Vegetable in both cooked and raw form
Eat Sufficiently—Fruits, Juices

Rice, Roti, Bread, cereals, noodles - Eat Enough

Total Calories

Total calories allowed to an individual will depend on the present weight and the targeted optimal weight.

Each serving in this Group contains 12 gms. of carbohydrates, 6 gms. of proteins and 1 gram of fat and gives approximately 80 calories.

Fats and oils

Each serving in the Fats and Oils Group contains 5 gms. of fat and gives 45 calories.

One serving is a teaspoon (5ml) of cooking oil.

Pulses and Dals

Each serving in the Group is about 25 gms. by weight if uncooked and about 1 cup cooked (thin, watery) or 1/2 cup cooked (thick).

Vegetables

More food should be eaten from this Food Group than from Groups.

Each serving in this group contains 5 gms. of carbohydrates, 2 gms. of proteins and gives approximately 28 calories.

For vegetables, one cup of raw leafy greens, three/quarters cup vegetable juice, or half a cup of chopped/cooked vegetables constitutes a serving.

Milk and milk based products

Each serving of skimmed milk and skimmed milk based foods contain 12 gms. of carbohydrates, 8 gms. of proteins and gives 80 calories.

Each serving of Whole Milk and Whole milk based products contains 12 gms. of carbohydrates, 8gms. of proteins, 8 gms. of fat and gives 150 calories.

Note

In the diet charts, milk servings are of the skimmed or toned milk variety unless stated otherwise.

For the milk group, a serving is one cup of milk or yoghurt or one and one half ounces of paneer.

One serving of food from the milk and yoghurt group is:

1 cup fat-free milk or 1 cup non-fat yoghurt
1 cup buttermilk

Meat

Each serving of food items in the Lean Meat Group (chicken/ fish) contains 7 gms. of proteins and 3gms. of fat and gives 55 calories.

Each serving of food items in the Medium Fat Meat Group (red meat) contains 7 gms. of proteins and 5 gms. of fats and gives 75 calories

Each serving of food items in the High Fat Meat Group (Red Meat) contains 7 gms. of proteins and 8 gms. of fats and gives 100 calories

Note

In the Diet Charts meat items are of the Lean Meat variety.

If meat items from the Medium Fat Meat group is eaten, you will have to substract half a serving of fats/Oils allowed in your diet.

If meat items from High Fat Meat group are eaten, you will have to substract one fat serving from the fat/oils servings allowed in your diet.

It is advisable to mostly choose items from the Lean Meat group. Foods from the other two groups, especially from the High Fat Meat group, should be eaten sparingly.

One serving in the Meat Group consists of items weighing approximately one ounce (30 gms.).

Examples of one serving of food from the Meat food group are:

one ounce cooked fish	one ounce cooked chicken	one ounces cooked ham burger

Cereals

The Cereal Group forms the base of the Pyramid and a large portion of your meal would consist of foods taken from this group.

Each serving in the Cereal Group contains 15 gms. of carbohydrates, 3 gms. of proteins, a trace of fat and gives about 80 calories.

Examples of one serving of food from this group are:

1 Slice of Bread, 1/2 cup rice, 1/2 cup cooked cereals 1 small baked potato

or

¾ cup dry flakes of cereal

Note

Very starchy vegetables such as potatoes, yam and corn are included in the Cereal List.

Select your calorie levels

How many calories should you be eating? This will depend on what your present weight is compared to what your ideal or optimal weight should be.

Measure your present weight and height and then use the BMI chart to see how your present weight compares to your optimal weight.

This will give you a good idea of the changes, if any, which you will need to make in your diet.

Optimal weight

Body mass index

Ideally, Body Mass Index (BMI) should be used to calculate optimal weight using the following formula:-

$$\text{BMI} = \frac{\text{Weight in kg.}}{\text{Height in metres}^2}$$

Care must be taken that the weight is not decreased below the desired weight, as a BMI of 18.5 signifies under-nutrition.

World Health Organisation Defines

Over weight as a Body Mass Index (BMI) of at least 25kg/m^2 and obesity as a BMI of at least 30 kg/m^2. Health risk rise progressively above BMI levels of 20-22 kg/m^2 in all population.

WHO recommends a general limit for waist circumference of 90 cms and 80 cms in men and women respectively.

Over weight and obesity lead to adverse metabolic effects on blood pressure, blood-sugar and insulin sensitivity.

Risks of coronary heart disease, ischemia, stroke and type 2 diabetes mellitus increase steadily with increasing body mass index

Body mass index is calculated by dividing weight in kilograms (kg) by square of height in metres (m)

BMI > 25 = over weight IDEAL BMI < 24

BMI - 25-29.9 = pre-obesity

BMI > 30 = obesity

Waist-hip (W-H) ratio

Recent evidence suggests that central obesity as judged by the Waist to Hip (W-H) ratio is important in diabetes and should be taken into consideration along with BMI.

A W-H ratio >0.95 in men and >0.85 in women denotes risk for the development of diabetes.

In the next pages you will find the body mass index calculator.

How to calculate your BMI?

First check your height (in inches-column on the left of the page) and your body weight (in pounds—mentioned in the box). You will be able to correspond your BMI which is mentioned on the top of the page.

Body mass index

Height (Inches)	19	20	21	22	23	24	25	26	27	28	29	30	31	32	33	34	35
	Body Weight (pounds)																
58	91	196	100	105	110	115	119	124	129	134	138	143	128	155	158	162	167
59	94	99	104	109	114	119	124	128	133	138	143	148	153	158	163	168	173
60	97	102	107	112	118	123	128	133	138	143	148	153	158	163	168	174	179
61	100	106	111	116	122	127	132	137	143	148	153	158	164	169	174	180	185
62	104	109	115	120	126	131	136	142	147	153	158	164	169	175	180	186	191
63	107	113	118	124	130	135	141	146	152	158	163	169	175	180	186	191	197
64	110	116	123	128	134	140	145	151	157	163	169	174	180	186	192	197	204
65	114	120	126	132	138	144	150	156	162	169	174	180	186	192	198	204	210
66	118	124	130	136	142	148	155	161	167	173	179	186	192	198	204	210	216
67	121	127	134	140	146	153	159	166	172	178	185	191	198	204	211	217	223
68	125	131	138	144	151	158	164	171	177	184	190	197	203	210	216	223	230
69	128	135	142	149	155	162	169	176	182	189	196	203	209	216	223	230	236
70	132	139	146	153	160	167	174	181	188	195	202	209	216	222	229	236	243
71	136	143	150	157	165	172	179	186	193	200	208	215	222	229	236	243	250
72	140	147	154	162	169	177	184	191	199	206	213	221	228	235	242	250	258
73	144	151	159	166	174	182	189	197	204	212	219	227	235	242	250	257	265
74	148	155	163	171	179	186	194	202	210	218	225	233	241	249	256	264	272
75	152	160	168	175	184	192	200	208	216	224	232	240	248	256	264	272	279
76	186	164	172	180	189	197	205	213	221	230	238	264	254	263	271	279	287

Body mass index

Height (Inches)	36	37	38	39	40	41	42	43	44	45	46	47	48	49	50	51	52	53	54
	Body Weight (pounds)																		
58	172	177	181	186	191	196	201	205	210	215	220	224	229	234	239	244	249	253	258
59	178	183	188	193	198	203	208	212	217	222	227	232	237	242	247	252	257	262	267
60	184	189	194	199	204	209	215	220	225	230	235	240	245	250	255	261	266	271	276
61	190	195	201	206	211	217	222	227	232	238	243	248	254	259	264	269	275	280	285
62	196	202	207	213	218	224	229	235	240	246	251	256	262	267	273	278	284	289	295
63	203	208	214	220	225	231	237	242	248	254	259	265	270	278	282	287	293	299	304
64	209	215	221	227	232	238	244	250	256	262	267	273	279	285	292	296	302	308	314
65	216	222	228	234	240	246	252	258	264	270	276	282	288	294	300	306	312	318	324
66	223	229	235	241	247	253	260	266	272	278	284	291	297	303	309	315	322	328	234
67	230	236	242	249	255	261	268	274	282	287	293	299	306	312	319	325	331	338	344
68	236	243	249	256	262	269	276	282	289	295	302	308	315	322	328	335	341	348	354
69	243	250	257	263	270	277	284	291	297	304	311	318	324	331	338	345	351	358	365
70	250	257	264	271	278	285	292	299	306	313	320	327	324	341	348	355	362	369	376
71	257	265	272	279	286	293	301	308	315	322	329	338	343	351	358	365	372	379	386
72	265	272	279	287	294	302	309	316	324	331	338	346	353	361	368	375	383	390	397
73	272	280	288	295	302	310	318	325	333	340	348	355	363	371	378	386	393	401	408
74	280	287	295	303	311	319	326	334	342	330	358	365	373	381	389	396	404	412	420
75	287	295	303	311	319	327	335	343	351	359	367	375	383	391	399	407	415	423	431
76	295	304	312	320	328	336	344	353	361	369	377	385	394	402	410	418	426	435	443

Judge Optimal body weight

Underweight	Normal weight	Overweight
May have to increase food intake to optimise weight	Continue same amount of food intake: may need to increase food intake to make up for calories lost through avoiding sugar.	Gradual decrease in amount if food normally eaten, if excessive, increase activity level also.

If you then find that you need to lose weight, you will have to decrease the total number of calories which you are taking.

Remember that 7700 calories is equivalent to one Kilogram of body weight.

In other words, in order to loose one kilogram of weight, you will have to have a negative balance of 7700 calories. In simple terms, your body must spend 7700 calories more than it takes in, in the form of food to lose this weight.

At first glance this seems to be a huge amount of calories, but don't be put off by this. Remember that most people who are overweight eat around 2500-3000 calories per day and more importantly, the weight loss is not done in a few days. In fact, one should strive to lose about 1.5 to 2 kilograms every month. So basically, we are talking about a negative calorie balance of around 12,000 to 15,000 calories in one month. This does not seem too much if you consider that the person who is overweight may be taking in almost 90,000 calories or more in a month!

A word of caution, please do not try and be over enthusiastic to loose weight very rapidly. Not only will this mean that you will have to drastically cut down your diet, and exercise rigorously, but such changes may not be good for you. Moreover, you can not continue this regime for a long period of time and this means that you might loose weight rapidly initially, but you will soon go back to your old schedule and regain the lost weight. Then after a while it is back to the rigid diet and exercise schedule. This has been well documented and is called the Yo-Yo phenomenon, where the weight goes up and down in cycles!

There may be some of you who may have optimal weight and therefore will not need to make too many changes to your present day diet except for some modifications such as direct sugar intake.

Some of you may be surprised to find that your weight is less than you should and especially if your BMI is lower than 18.5-19 then you should slightly increase your diet in order to gain some weight. Here again, increase your calories slowly and aim for a slow and gradual weight gain. But, you should not gorge on sweets! The basic principles of a diabetic diet still hold true.

To sum up

(1) Measure your weight and height.
(2) Estimate your optimal body weight.
(3) Decide what changes in your weight you will need to make.
(4) Calculate the calories intake needed to maintain your present weight with the diet you eat and your activity levels.
(5) Estimate the calories requirements to gradually reach optimal weight.

For Weight Loss—Healthy Eating Tips

1. Use methods like steaming, baking, grilling, boiling etc. and cooking in a small amount of oil rather than deep-frying. Use more of Non-Stick cookwares.
2. Always heat oil thoroughly before sauteing food, since cold oil is absorbed more readily.
3. Low fat foods don't have to be tasteless and boring—so transform your low fat cooking into exotic dishes with herbs and spices.
4. Always eat slowly—Don't Rush. Chew every mouthful of food deliberately. It helps your body to feel full, so that you'll be less likely to over eat.
5. Before cooking fish or chicken, skin off all the extra fat, then just brush with little oil.
6. Eat slowly. Brain takes about 20 minutes to get the message that you are full.
7. Don't leave serving platters on the table when the meal is over. It will encourage second helping and over eating.

8. Party should not be an excuse for eating wrong foods. You can have healthy meals there as well. Keep your diet plan in mind and choose the foods sensibly. Go easier on Fried, Paneer Dishes, Non-Veg items, Sweets and Alcohol. Rather have more of salads and vegetables.
9. Explain your eating goals to your family and friends. Ask them not to offer second helping or urge you to eat more.
10. Remodel your old recipes and try to use measuring cups and spoons.
11. Use only low fat dairy products curd, milk etc.
12. For salads use a low fat dressing with olive oil or low fat curd, orange juice or lemon, herbs etc. can be used in place of mayonaise.
13. Try to reduce the amount of salt use in cooking and at table. Instead flavor the foods with lemon juice, herbs, spices of mustard for a healthier and tastier food.
14. Experiment by using less sugar when you bake. Recipe such as Fruit Cake can be made without added sugar. Artificial sweeteners can be added instead.
15. Avoid Refined flours like Maida and Sweet Foods, Jams, Chocolates, Cakes, Sweet Cream etc.

Facts About Diet

Food and Nutrition

Good health is a state of complete physical, mental and social well-being and not merely the absence of disease. According to World Health Organization, good health is not just an absence of disease or illness but it involves physical, psychological and social well-being of an individual.

The 3 main components of a healthy lifestyle are:

1. Regular exercise—Exercise can be defined as physical activity that is a planned, structured movement of the body designed to enhance physical fitness.
2. Balanced diet—Eating healthy is also an important component of a healthy lifestyle. (*to be discussed separately*)
3. Stress management—The definition of stress management then, is basically that it is the emotional and physical strain that is caused by our response to pressures from the outside world. This strain varies in terms of severity and impact from person to person, as each person handles stress differently and responds differently to separate stressors as well, stressors being the factors in our lives that cause us the stress.

Stress is the body's way of responding to any kind of demand, both by good and bad experiences. When people feel stressed by something that is going on around them, their bodies end up reacting to this by releasing chemicals into the blood, and these chemicals give people more energy and strength, but can also have a turnaround effect and end up making them sad or depressed.

Regardless of how severe your stress is or how long you have been dealing with it for, if you notice any symptoms that are a result of this stress, it is very important that you get yourself to see your doctor as soon as you possibly can. Your physician can help you to define your particular stresses and prescribe medications and therapies that can help you on your info on stress management.

Nutrition: The science of foods, nutrients and other substances therein, their action, interaction and balance in relation to health and disease.

Eating well is vital for a healthy and active life. When the nutritional requirements of an individual are not met, it may lead to a condition known as *Malnutrition.*

Malnutrition is a broad term commonly used as an alternative to undernutrition but technically it also refers to overnutrition.

People are malnourished if their diet does not provide adequate calories and protein for growth and maintenance or they are unable to fully utilize the food they eat due to illness (undernutrition).

They are also malnourished if they consume too many calories (overnutrition).

Development of Undernutrition

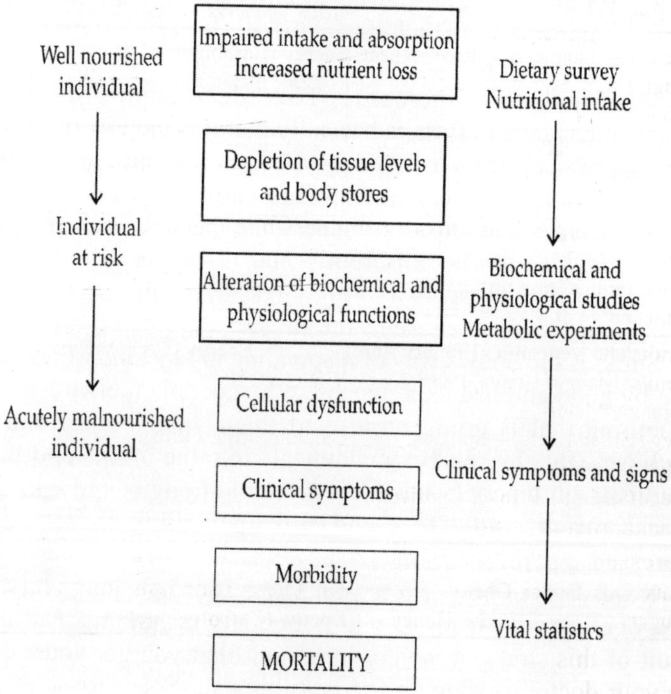

How to overcome Malnutrition

- Balanced diet
  — small and frequent meals
  — eat or drink nutritional supplement
- Medication
- Consulting health care team
- Positive approach

Balanced diet: The diet which contains different types of foods in such quantities and proportions that the needs for all the nutrients are adequately met.

To meet an individual's balanced diet, it is important to understand the concept of various foods that make diet plan or a balanced meal so that each component is rightly distributed and understood. The "Five Food Group System" helps in defining balanced diet components. The distribution is as follows:

Food Groups	*Main Nutrients*
1. Cereals—(staple diet) Rice, Wheat, Ragi, Bajra, Maize, Jowar, Riceflakes	Energy (Carbohydrate) Protein, B-complex vitamins, Iron, Fibre
2. Pulses and Legumes (veg. protein) All dals, Soyabean, Rajmah, Cowpea, Peas, Beans	Energy (Carbohydrate) Protein, B-complex vitamins, Iron, Calcium, Fibre
3. Milk and Milk products, (animal protein) Milk, Curds, Paneer Meat (animal protein) Chicken, Fish, Egg, Mutton	Protein, Fat, Calcium, Vitamin B2,
4. Fruits and Vegetables (dietary fibre) Fruits: Mango, Guava, Papaya, Orange, Melon Veg (Green Leafy)—Spinach, Methi, Bathua Veg (Others)—Brinjal, Capsicum, Cauliflower	Energy (Carbohydrate) Vitamin C, Fibre Vitamin B Complex, Calcium, Iron, Fibre
5. Fats and Sugars (calories/energy) Fats: Oils, Butter, Ghee Sugars : Sugar, Jaggary, Honey	Fat, Energy (calories) Energy (Carbohydrate)

Importance of food group system

1. **Tool for nutritional assessment and screening**—a brief diet history system can disclose inadequacies of nutrient from any of the 5 groups. This information can be the first clue for the possibility of the subject may be at the risk of developing nutritional deficiency.
2. **Tool for nutritional counselling**—the dietary history based on 5 food group system allows a health team to counsel a patient about nutrition i.e. a diet plan.
3. **Explaining therapeutic diets to a patient**—therapeutic (***Treatment and care to combat disease***) diets are scientifically based on nutrient composition and food groups which can be used in menu planning.

Generally, nutrients are divided into two classes: macro nutrients and micro nutrients.

Macro (major) nutrients are required daily in large quantities. They include proteins, fats, carbohydrates and water.

Micro (minor) nutrients are required daily in small quantities. They include vitamins and trace minerals that enable the body to use macro nutrients.

Nutritional components of food.

Macro nutrients—carbohydrates, proteins, fats, water.

Micro nutritients—vitamins and minerals

The nutritional requirements of all individuals vary from one another depending upon age, gender, physical activity, physiological stress or condition (e.g. pregnancy or lactation).

Recommended Dietary Allowance (RDA)

- Average daily nutrient intake level that meets the needs of nearly all (97-98%) healthy people in a particular life stage and gender group.
- RDA are given for different groups: adults, infants, children, pregnant and lactating women.

- Takes into account individual variation in nutrient needs and availability of nutrients which may vary from diet to diet.

Meal Planning: Meal planning is planning what you are going to serve for a certain amount of time, could be a week, could be a day, and could be a month. It involves organizing the ingredients and recipes.

Principles of Meal Planning

- Meeting nutritional requirements—already discussed.
- Fulfil family needs—ensure that diet does not vary according to each member in family, rather it meets everyones needs when put together. For e.g. it is not advisable to plan 5 different kinds of meals for 5 members in breakfast or any meal, it is important to understand the distribution of macro and micro nutrients and then plan in common.
- Save time and energy—meals planned should not be time consuming.
- Economics—meal planning also involves meeting the financial condition of the individual or family. For e.g. if protein intake is not sufficient and the person can make changes in diet, it is not advisable to add supplements replacing diet and adding extra cost burden.
- Provide maximum nutrients.
- Likes and dislikes (veg./non-veg)—it is very important to meet the likes and dislikes of the person. For e.g. Roti and dal cannot be prescribed to a person who is living in south India for all the meals.
- Variety—ensure that all nutrients are a part of diet plan, therefore, adding variety, colour, flavour and most important there is no monotony in the plan.
- Satiety—it means distributing the meals in such a way that the person should not feel starved or dissatisfied with the portion size after the meal, i.e. meal should give a feeling of fullness but not over loading.

Notes on Macro Nutrients

Carbohydrates, proteins, and fats supply 90 per cent of the dry weight of the diet and 100 per cent of its energy. As sources of energy, carbohydrates, proteins, and fats are interchangeable in proportion to their energy content. The energy content is 4 calories in a gram of carbohydrate or protein and 9 calories in a gram of fat. However, these nutrients differ in how quickly they supply energy; carbohydrates are the quickest, and fats are the slowest.

Carbohydrates, proteins, and fats are digested in the intestine, where they are broken down into their basic units: carbohydrates into sugars, proteins into amino acids, and fats into fatty acids and glycerol. The body uses these basic units to build substances it needs for growth, maintenance, and activity (including other carbohydrates, proteins, and fats).

***Carbohydrates*:** Energy producing compound that makes up about half of our food intake .1 Gm of carbohydrate = 4 Kcal. These are a group of organic compounds, including sugars, starches and fibre.

Depending on the size of the molecule, carbohydrates may be **simple or complex.**

Simple carbohydrates are various forms of sugar. Because they are small molecules; they can be broken down by the body quickly and are the quickest source of energy.

Monosaccharide ("mono" = one + "saccharide" = sugar) is the simplest form of carbohydrate. Glucose, Fructose and Galactose are monosaccharides.

- ➢ **Glucose** is the chief end product of digestion of disaccharides and polysaccharides.
- It is found in sweet fruits such as grapes, berries and oranges and in some vegetables such as sweet corns and carrots.
- It is the form of carbohydrate circulating in the blood and it is utilized by the cell for energy.
- ➢ **Fructose** is also known as fruit sugar
- It is found in honey, ripe fruits and some vegetables
- ➢ **Galactose** is produced by the hydrolysis of lactose.

Food sources of simple carbohydrates include sugar, honey, refined flour, fruit juices, soft drink, cakes, cookies, chapatti, idli, noodles, plain rice etc.

Disaccharide ("di" = two + "saccharide" = sugar): made up of 2 single sugar units linked together

SUCROSE = GLUCOSE + FRUCTOSE

(Table Sugar) found in cane, beet root

LACTOSE = GLUCOSE + GALACTOSE

(Milk sugar)

MALTOSE = GLUCOSE + GLUCOSE

(present in beer and malted breakfast cereals)

Complex carbohydrates are composed of long strings of simple carbohydrates. Because complex carbohydrates are larger molecules than simple carbohydrates, they are slower sources of energy.

➢ Polysaccharide (more than one sugar): they don't taste sweet
  - Starch—it is the storage form of carbohydrates in plants.
  - Glycogen—it is the storage form of carbohydrates in humans and animals.
  - Fibre—it is the indigestible form of carbohydrate, provide structure to plant.
  - Dextrin—it is the breakdown product of long chains of starch during digestion.

Complex carbohydrates occur in wheat products (such as breads and pastas), other grains (such as rye and corn), beans, and root vegetables (such as potatoes).

The body stores very small amounts of excess energy as carbohydrates. The liver stores some as glycogen, a complex carbohydrate that the body can easily and rapidly convert to energy. Muscles also store glycogen, which they use during periods of intense exercise. The amount of carbohydrates stored as glycogen provides almost a day's worth of calories.

Functions of Carbohydrates

Main source of energy

- Excess of calories consumed in the form of carbohydrates are stored as fat in the adipose tissue
- Protein Sparing Effect
- Dietary fibre help relieve constipation
- Increases satiety (feeling of fullness)
- Delays glucose absorption
- Reduces serum cholesterol

Most authorities recommend that about 50 to 55 per cent of the total daily calories should consist of carbohydrates.

Fibre

Include all parts of plant food that body can't digest or absorb. Also known as roughage or bulk.

Dietary fibre can be classified in 2 forms:

1. Soluble fibre
2. Insoluble fibre

Soluble Fibre	*Insoluble Fibre*
It is the edible portion of plant foods, resistant to digestion and absorption in small intestine. While passing through large intestine (colon) partial or total fermentation occurs due to the action of colonic bacteria. It dissolves in water to form a gel like substance.	It is made up of the structural material of the cell wall of plant foods. It does not dissolve rather soaks up adding bulk to the stool, soften the stool and increases the transit time through the intestinal tract.
It lowers total and LDL (bad) cholesterol, reducing risk of heart disease. Regulates blood sugar levels in people with diabetes.	It promotes regular bowel movement and prevents constipation. Removes toxic waste material from the intestines faster. Gives satiety (a feeling of fullness), therefore, helps in weight loss.
Found in pulp of fruits, legumes, oats and greens.	Found in skin of various fruits, green vegetables, wheat bran.

Diabetes and Gastroparesis

- Gastroparesis, also called delayed gastric emptying, is a disorder in which the stomach takes too long to empty its contents.
- It often occurs in people with type 1 diabetes or type 2 diabetes.
- Gastroparesis happens when nerves to the stomach are damaged or stop working. The vagus nerve controls the movement of food through the digestive tract. If the vagus nerve is damaged, the muscles of the stomach and intestines do not work normally, and the movement of food is slowed or stopped.
- Diabetes can damage the vagus nerve if blood glucose level remains high over a long period of time. High blood glucose causes chemical changes in nerves and damages the blood vessels that carry oxygen and nutrients to the nerves.

Signs and Symptoms of Gastroparesis

- Heartburn
- Nausea
- Vomiting of undigested food
- An early feeling of fullness when eating
- Weight loss
- Abdominal bloating
- Erratic blood glucose levels
- Lack of appetite

These symptoms may be mild or severe, depending on the severity of disease.

Points to remember for dietary advise for Gastroparesis

√ Eat smaller, more frequent meal.
√ Low insoluble fibre foods.

- √ Low fat diet.
- √ Eat and drink all foods and beverages while sitting.
- √ Solid foods are often better tolerated earlier in the day with a switch to semi-solid or liquid meals later in the day.

Glycemic Index

- ➢ Glycemic Index is the ability of carbohydrates to raise the blood glucose.
- ➢ It is a quantitative assessment of foods based blood glucose level after a meal.
- ➢ Per cent of the response to an equivalent CHO portion of a reference food.
- ➢ Reference food is white bread with GI set at 100.

Factors affecting Glycemic Index

- **Size:** Grains that are in their original form like whole wheat and barley have a lower GI than other forms of these substances such as refined flours
- **Processing:** Pounding, mixing, grinding (processing) decreases the particle size
  e.g. Whole wheat→broken wheat (dalia)→semolina (suji)→refined wheat flour (maida)
- **Fibre content:** Fibre slows down the emptying of bowels.

Glycemic Load

- Glycemic load of a particular food is the product of the glycemic index of the food and the amount of carbohydrate in a serving.
- By summing the glycemic load contributed by individual foods, the overall glycemic load of a meal or the whole diet can be calculated.

How Glycemic Load is Calculated

The formula for calculating glycemic load is simple. Multiply the GI value of a food by the amount of carbohydrate per serving and divide the result by 100.

An apple has a GI value of 40

1. A serving (medium size apple) contains 15 grams of carbohydrate, (GI = 40)
   The glycemic load of an apple is: (40 × 15) = 600 divided by 100 = 600/100 = 6

Mixed fruit jam has a GI value of 51

2. 1 tsp of jam (GI = 51) : (51 × 5 g jam)/100 = 2.5

GI and GL for Common Foods

Food	*GI*	*Serving Size*	*Net Carbs*	*GL*
Bean sprouts	25	1 cup	4	1
Grapefruit	25	½ large	11	3
Pizza	30	2 slices (med)	42	13
Low fat yoghurt	33	1 cup	47	16
Apples	38	1 medium	16	6
Spaghetti	42	1 cup	38	16
Carrots	47	1 large	5	2
Oranges	48	1 medium	12	6
Banana	52	1 large	27	14
Potato chips	54	4 oz	55	30
Snickers Bar	55	1 bar	64	35
Brown rice	55	1 cup	42	23
Honey	55	1 tbsp	17	9
Oatmeal	58	1 cup	21	12
Icecream	61	1 cup	16	10
Macaroni and cheese	64	1 serving	47	30
Raisins	64	1 small box	32	20
White rice	64	1 cup	52	33
Sugar (sucrose)	68	1 tbsp	12	8
White bread	100	1 slice	14	14
Watermelon	72	1 cup	11	8
Popcorn	72	2 cups	10	7
Baked potato	85	1 medium	33	28
Glucose	100	(50 g)	50	50

GI's of 55 or below are considered low, and 70 or above are considered high
GL's of 10 or below are considered low, and 20 or above are considered high.

Points to remember

- √ Eat at regular times
- √ Choose a variety of foods from all food groups
- √ Limit simple sugars
- √ Include food sources from complex carbohydrates in every main meal
- √ It is not only the quality (GI) but also the quantity (GL) of carbohydrates that is important in the meal plan.

Proteins: The word "protein" is derived from the Greek word "proteios", which means primary or holding first place. The way the name suggests this group of components are the most important cell constituent. Protein is present in all cells of the body. It is present in variable level in different tissues of the body like muscles contain about 20 per cent whereas in blood plasma it is 7 per cent.

Functions of Dietary Protein

1. Proteins are necessary structural integrity of cells and growth of the body.
2. They are required for the formation of enzymes, digestive juices, haemoglobin and hormones.
3. Required for the protection of the body against infection.
4. Proteins help in the transport of oxygen and nutrients.
5. Protein is required for tissue repair.
6. Needed for the production of milk proteins during lactation.
7. To replace the daily loss of body proteins.

Proteins are also a source of energy (this is not desirable because if proteins are utilized for energy, then it will not be able to provide protection against infections, growth and repair which may lead to increased susceptibility to infections). Each gram of protein provides 4 kcal.

Therefore, when carbohydrates constitute to about 50 per cent of the dietary intake it is referred to as Protein Sparing action where in proteins are not utilized for giving energy to various cells of body.

Therefore, it is essential to have a balanced diet with all nutrients in required amounts as per the individual.

Each protein in the body is tailored for a specific need, proteins are not interchangeable. Body cannot directly use proteins found in food. Dietary protein is broken down into its constituent amino acids, which the body then uses to build the different specific proteins it needs. It is the amino acids rather than protein that are the essential nutrients.

Amino Acids are the chemical units or "building blocks" of the body that make up proteins. There are 22 amino acids found in plant and animal proteins.

Essential Amino Acids: (9)

These cannot be synthesized in the body, hence have to be obtained from the food.

Histidine, Isoleucine, Leucine, **Lysine, Methionine,** Phenylalanine, Threonine, Tryptophan, Valine.

Non-Essential Amino Acid : (11)

These can be synethesized in the body, hence need not be obtianed from the diet.

Alanine, Arginine, Aspartic Acid, Cystine, Glutamine, Glycine, Ornithine, Proline, Serine, Taurine, Tyrosine.

Types of Protein

Dietary protein can be classified in 2 forms:

1. Complete or Class 1 protein
2. Incomplete or Class 2 protein

Complete/Class 1 Protein	*Incomplete/Class 2 Protein*
√ Provide all EAA in adequate amounts and proportion seeded by the body for growth and tissue maintenance	√ These are deficient in one or more EAA
√ Totally used by body and very little waste is left	√ Not completely used by the body and produce more waste products
√ Animal protein	√ Plant protein
√ Fish, chicken, eggs, meat and dairy products	√ Legumes, pulses, cereals, soybeans and nuts

➢ ***Nitrogen Balance:*** The difference between the dietary intake of nitrogen (mainly protein) and its excretion (as urea and other waste products)

Nitrogen Balance = N (intake) – N (excretion)
Healthy adults excrete the same amount as is ingested, and so are in Nitrogen equilibrium.

Nitrogen Equilibrium – Intake = Excretion
Positive Nitrogen Balance is a condition where the intake of protein increases its excretion or output.

Intake > Excretion
For e.g.: Pregnancy, lactation, growth, adequate protein intake

Negative Nitrogen Balance is a condition where the intake of protein is less than its excretion or output.

Excretion > Intake
For e.g. Malnourishment, burns, fever, injury, post-surgery, starvation, Inadequate protein intake.

Protein quality : The most important function of dietary protein is to maintain body tissues and promote growth. Proteins differ in their capacity to maintain body tissue and promote growth. It depends upon the protein "quality".

Protein quality depends upon:

1. Whether or not the dietary protein supplies all 9 essential amino acids.
2. The ratio or the proportion of amino acids in the dietary proteins as compared to that needed in the body.
3. Digestibility: A measure of the amount of amino acids absorbed from a given dietary protein.

Improving protein quality **:** In general, **plant proteins are of lower quality** than animal proteins, and plants also provide **less protein per gram of food.**

Deficiency of an amino acid in one food item can be compensated for by combining it with another food item which has it in adequate amounts. This is known as **Mutual Supplementation.**

Complementary proteins provide all essential amino acids in quantities needed to support health.

Limiting amino acid: The amino acid that is found in shortest supply relative to the amount needed for the protein synthesis by the body. The most common limiting amino acids are:

Lysine → Grains

Methionine → Beans and Legumes

1 **Cereal Protein + Pulse Protein**

Example: Idli or Dosa with sambhar, Dhokla

A combination of cereal and pulse in the ratio of 5 : 1 has been found to be given an optimum combination.

2. **Plant Protein + Animal Protein**

Example: Dahi vada, Rice kheer, Curd rice

***Points to remember*:** In general, proteins of uncooked vegetable foods (esp. pulses) are less digestible than those of animal foods.

Some pulses used in food contain chemical constituents having toxic properties.

Trypsin inhibitors proteins that inhibit the activity of Trypsin in the gut and interfere with the digestibility of dietary proteins and reduce their utilization. These are destroyed on cooking.

Soybean has a powerful trypsin inhibitor which is destroyed by dry roasting for 15-20 minutes. Therefore, cooking and heat treatment improves the digestibility of protein in several foods.

Protein deficiency: Lack of dietary protein may lead to following conditions:

- Stunted growth in children
- Muscle wasting
- Increased susceptibility to infection.
- Poor wound healing
- Anemia
- Edema

***RDA of Protein*:** Average daily protein requirement of an Indian adult is **1g/kg present body weight/day**

***Fats*:** Fats are organic compounds that are made up of carbon, hydrogen, and oxygen; they are the most concentrated source of energy in foods. Fats belong to a group of substances called lipids. Fats come in liquid or solid form. All fats are combinations of saturated and unsaturated fatty acids. Fat provides 9 calories per gram, more than twice the number provided by carbohydrates or protein.

***Functions of Fats*:** The functions of fats are as follows:

- Fat is the concentrated source of energy.
  1gm fat = 9 Kcal
- It is stored in the fat cells within the adipose (fat) tissue. Body fat provides the most important reservoir of stored energy as adipose tissue. Even in a person who is not overweight, body fat still makes up about 10 per cent of their body weight. From a survival standpoint, this is absolutely critical, since in periods of low food availability or during a famine situation, a person must live off his/her stored body fat or perish.
- Fat is a fairly poor conductor of heat, body fat in the subcutaneous tissues (under the skin) acts as insulation, and tends to prevent loss of body heat.

- Fat, in the form of structural body fat, provides important protection for the vital internal organs.
- These protective deposits are the last to be drawn on for energy supplies when energy in the diet is inadequate.
- It helps in transportation and use of fat soluble vitamins A, D, E, and K. Without fat in the diet, those vitamins would not be able to function. This would result in severe problems with eyesight, skin, nail formation, blood clotting, kidney function, bone growth and repair, reproductive functions, and cellular energy.

Classification of fats: Fats can be classified on the basis of heir visibility and chemical structure.

Visibility	*Visible fats*	*Invisible fats*
Chemical Structure	Saturated fats Medium chain triglycerides	Unsaturated fats (a) Monounsaturated fats (b) Polyunsaturated fats

Classification of Fats depending on visibility

Visible fats	*Invisible fats*
They are visible to the naked eye. It includes all the fats and oils that are used for cooking. For e.g.: Butter, ghee, oils, vanaspati or dalda, processed cheese.	They are not visible to the naked eye but add to the calories in the food. All foods contain invisible fats in varying amounts. For e.g.: Cereals, pulses, dairy products, nuts, oilseeds, eggs, meat.

Classification of fats depending on chemical structure

1a. Saturated fats—They are solid/semi-solid at room temperature, with the exception of certain oils. They are usually from animal sources.

E.g.: Ghee, butter, cheese, whole milk and products, coconut oil, palm oil (plant source).

They increases LDL (bad) cholesterol and reduces HDL (good) cholesterol and increases plasma triglycerides (TG) levels as well.

b. **Medium Chain Triglycerides**—These are saturated fatty acids, but with a slight difference in their structure. MCTs are more readily hydrolyzed and absorbed than conventional food fat. They require less enzymes and bile acids for digestion than conventional food fat. These are of use in patients suffering from pancreatic and liver disorders.

   E.g.: Coconut oil, palm oil, butter and commercial products.

3. **Unsaturated fats**—These are liquid at room temperature. These are commonly found in vegetables, nuts, and seeds. They help lower blood cholesterol level but amount consumed needs to be checked.

   There are two types: mono-unsaturated fatty acids (MUFAs) and polyunsaturated fatty acids (PUFAs)—(a) Omega 3 (b) Omega 6.

Mono-unsaturated fatty acids—Mono-unsaturated oils are liquid at room temperature but start to solidify at refrigerator temperatures. They are less susceptible to oxidation. They have favourable effect on blood lipids when consumed in moderate amounts. Helps decrease the level of LDL (bad) cholesterol.

For e.g.: olive oil, groundnut oil, rice bran oil, sesame oil, red palm oil.

Poly-unsaturated fatty acids—Poly-unsaturated oils are liquid at room temperature and in refrigerator as well. They easily combine with oxygen in the air to become rancid.

It includes omega 6 (linoleic) and omega 3 (linolenic) fatty acids, also called as **essential fatty acids**—The body cannot synthesize the essential fatty acids. They must be consumed in the diet.

Sources of Omega 6 fatty acids are corn oil, safflower oil, sesame oil (til), sunflower oil, soybean oil and cottonseed oil.

Sources of Omega 3 fatty acids are fish, fish oils, walnuts, flaxseeds, green leafy vegetables, soybean, rajma, and cowpea.

Studies have shown that *"Omega-3s" from fish are highly polyunsaturated fatty acids that lower triglycerides, reduce abnormal heart rhythms, reduce blood pressure by small but significant amounts, and improve blood clotting regulation.*

- ➢ Omega-3 fatty acids may be particularly beneficial for overweight people with hypertension who are on weight loss diets. Dr. Trevor Mori and colleagues at the University of Western Australia recently showed that people on a weight loss diet that included fat-rich fish daily had improved glucose and insulin metabolism.
- ➢ Japanese, who also consume large amounts of fish, have much lower rates of heart disease and diabetes than Americans.

The recommended ratio of omega 6 : omega 3 in diet is 4 : 1. Therefore, the oils that meet this recommendation are the preferred ones in the diet.

Blood cholesterol: Cholesterol is a fat like substance in the blood. It is made in liver and we also get cholesterol from certain foods in our diet. Too much cholesterol can build up in arteries over a long period of time. Hypercholesterolemia is the term used for high levels of blood cholesterol. It can cause heart attacks and stroke.

There are 2 sources of cholesterol in our body.

1. **ENDOGENOUS cholesterol** is what our body makes (75%).
2. **EXOGENOUS cholesterol** is that which comes from diet (25%)
   E.g. meat, poultry, fish egg yolk, butter, cheese and full cream milk and its products.
   Note: cholesterol is present only in animal foods

More about cholesterol—Lipoproteins are tiny spherical particles which circulate in the blood. They contain cholesterol, fat, and protein in varying amounts depending on where they are produced in the body and on the jobs they are directed to perform.

Abnormalities of the amounts or kinds of lipoproteins in blood can cause increased risk of atherosclerosis in the coronary arteries (leading to heart attack, angina or coronary pain, or sudden death) and atherosclerosis in many other arteries in the body. **Atherosclerosis is sometimes referred to as hardening or narrowing of the arteries, cholesterol deposition, or arterial blockage.** Other risk factors such as smoking, high blood pressure, diabetes, and sedentary lifestyle also contribute to the development of atherosclerosis. The risk from lipoprotein abnormalities can be especially severe, if a very high elevation of one type of lipoprotein is present, or if several lipoprotein abnormalities are found together in one person.

The total cholesterol level measures blood cholesterol in all lipoproteins combined. More specific measurements are LDL and HDL cholesterol.

Low Density Lipoproteins (LDL) perform the task of moving cholesterol from the liver to sites where it is used in other tissues. An increased level of total cholesterol in blood usually indicates high LDL cholesterol, since most of the total cholesterol is normally found in LDL. LDL is sometimes called the "bad" cholesterol, since some of the LDL particles enter the walls of arteries, where they form harmful cholesterol deposits. The higher the level of LDL cholesterol in blood, the more likely a person will develop coronary or other atherosclerotic disease.

High Density Lipoproteins (HDL) carry approximately one-fourth of the total amount of cholesterol in blood. Studies have shown that persons who have more of their blood cholesterol in HDL, as opposed to other lipoproteins, will have fewer heart attacks and coronary deaths. One of the functions of HDL is reverse cholesterol transport—that is, the transport of cholesterol from body tissues back to the liver. These facts suggest that the HDL cholesterol level can serve as a rough measure of the blood's ability to regulate (and reduce) the cholesterol content of body tissues. Cholesterol in HDL has been called the "good cholesterol".

Body fat is triglyceride. Certain lipoproteins (chylomicrons and Very Low Density Lipoproteins—VLDL) perform the job of transporting fat in the blood. The triglyceride in these lipoproteins comes from both body fat and dietary fat. Triglyceride is eventually broken down into fatty acids, which are the major fuel used by the body to produce movement and heat and to energize other chemical processes. High levels of triglyceride-rich lipoproteins are generally associated with increased coronary risk.

Trans fatty acids : Trans fatty acids are the fats produced by heating liquid vegetable oil in the presence of hydrogen. The process is known as hydrogenation. They are used in commercial baked goods and for cooking in most restaurants and fast-food chains. They raise LDL and lower HDL. The sources of trans fats in the diet are Bread, biscuits, pastries, puffs, vanaspati, margarine, commercially fried foods like french fries.

Dietary approaches for dealing with increased cholesterol

The Step I and Step II diets were created by the National Heart, Lung, and Blood Association's National Cholesterol Education Programme (NCEP). The American Heart Association endorsed them. Both diets were designed to reduce risk of cardiovascular disease by reducing high blood cholesterol levels.

Recommendation	*Step 1 diet*	*Step 2 diet*
Total fat	< 30% total calories	< 30% total calories
Saturated fat	< 10% total calories	< 7% total calories
MUFA	10-15% total calories	10-15% total calories
PUFA	< 10% total calories	< 10% total calories
Cholesterol	< 300 mg/day	< 200 mg/day

For people at high risk or who are known to suffer from heart disease, AHA has adopted the Therapeutic Lifestyle Changes (TLC) diet. This is the "next generation" of the Step II diet recommended in May 2001. That's when the NCEP released new guidelines for cholesterol management in its Third Report of the Expert Panel on Detection, Evaluation, and Treatment of High Blood Cholesterol in Adults.

Nutrient—Recommended Intake as Per cent of Total Calories:

- **Total Fat**—25–35 per cent
- **Saturated Fat**—Less than 7 per cent
- **Poly-unsaturated Fat**—Up to 10 per cent
- **Mono-unsaturated Fat**—Up to 20 per cent
- **Carbohydrate**—50-60 per cent of total calories
- **Protein**—Approximately 15 per cent
- **Cholesterol**—Less than 200 mg per day
- **Total Calories**—Balance energy intake and expenditure to maintain desirable body weight and prevent weight gain.

Role of fat in the diet

1. **SOURCE OF ENERGY:** Fat is the most concentrated source of energy in the diet. **1g of Fat = 9 kcal**
2. **SATIETY VALUE:** Fat tends to leave the stomach relatively slowly. It is released from the stomach 3.5 hrs after a meal depending on the size and composition of the meal. This prolonged stay in the stomach helps to delay the onset of hugner and so contributes to a feeling of satiety after a meal.
3. **PALATABILITY:** The presence of fat in food or its addition to food is responsible for much of the texture and flavour of food.

Recommendations by ADA

Recommendations		*For Diabetes Patients*
Total cholesterol		<160 mg/dl
LDL cholesterol		<70 mg/dl
HDL cholesterol	Men	>40 mg/dl
	Women	>50 mg/dl
Triglycerides		<150 mg/dl

MICRO NUTRIENTS

A substance, such as a vitamin or mineral, that is essential in minute amounts for the proper growth and metabolism of a living organism.

Vitamins

Although vitamins are necessary to maintain good health, they are neither sources of energy, nor significant contributors to the substance of the body. They act principally as regulators of metabolic processes. In general, none of them can be formed in the body—except niacin and vitamins A, D, and K. For those who are in relatively good health, adequate levels of the essential vitamins can be obtained through well-balanced diets.

Types of Vitamins

Water-Soluble

- soluble in water
- not stored in appreciable amounts
- regular consumption necessary
- excreted in the urine
- toxicity rare

  e.g. B-complex Vitamins and Vitamin C

Fat-Soluble

- soluble in fat
- absorbed and transported with dietary lipids
- significant amounts stored in the liver
- can result in toxicity
- e.g. Vitamin A, D, E, K

Water-Soluble Vitamins:

- B-Complex Vitamins: These include the following:
  √ Thiamine (vitamin B1)
  √ Riboflavin (vitamin B2)
  √ Niacin
  √ Pantothenic acid
  √ Pyriodoxine (vitamin B6)
  √ Biotin
  √ Folic acid
  √ Vitamin B12

All B-complex vitamins play an important part of key reactions of the metabolic processes in the body. They help in the conversion of food (CHO_4, proteins, fats) to energy; hence their requirements are energy-related.

Below is a table enlisting the food sources of important vitamins along with the causes of losses of these vitamins from the food.

Vitamin	*Major Food Sources*	*Causes of Losses*
Thiamine (B1)	Yeast, liver, cereal grains, nuts	Milling, refining, heat, excessive washing, baking, vigorous boiling, dehydration, overcooking, use of cooking soda
Riboflavin (B2)	Meat and dairy products, eggs, green leafy vegetables, soyabean	Use of baking soda, sun drying, cooking/boiling in excess water, milling of rice and wheat
Niacin	Meat, peanuts, dairy products, eggs, fish, whole grains, legumes	Grain processing
Pyridoxine (B6)	Whole grain foods (esp. wheat), meats, veg, nuts	
Folic acid	Green leafy veg, organ meats, oranges (Bio-availability is 25-50%)	Easily oxidised during storage, cooking, processing at high temperatures.
Vitamin B12	Seafood, meat and meat products, fish, eggs. Strict vegetarians more prone to deficiency	Pasteurization and evaporation of milk

Vitamin C

Vitamin C (ascorbic acid) is a water-soluble vitamin important in the synthesis of collagen (necessary for wound healing) and in the maintenance of healthy gums and teeth. It is abundant in most fresh fruit and vegetables.

Some important functions of vitamin C are:

- **Antioxidant:** Exposure to drugs, environmental pollutants and stress results in the formation of oxidative agents in the body (oxidative stress). Vitamin C converts these oxidizing agents to harmless substances that can be excreted. It can combine with and scavenge all these free radicals and thus protect the body from damage.
- **Absorption of Iron and Calcium:** Vitamin C helps keep iron and calcium in soluble forms thus enhancing their absorption. Hence, a source of vitamin C should always accompany an iron or calcium rich dish.

Sources: Include citrus fruits like amla, orange, guava; green leafy vegetables (drumstick leaves, spinach); tomatoes, capsicum; sprouted pulses. Animal foods **DO NOT** contain vit C. Raw fresh foods are better sources of vit C than cooked foods.

Vitamin C is easily destroyed by oxidation, light, alkali and heat. Some of the common causes of losses of vitamin C are:

- Removal of skin/peel of fruits/vegetables will cause vit C to leach into the water used for cooking.
- Cutting food into small pieces and then cooking, increases losses due to increased surface area exposed to water and heat. Hence, cook whole.
- Use of copper cooking vessels destroys the vitamin.
- Use of large amount of water.
- Use of cooking soda.

Vitamin A

It exists in 2 forms; Retinol form is present in animal foods and beta carotene is present in plant foods. Beta-carotene is a pigment in vegetables that gives them their yellow, orange or red colour. Once consumed, it is slowly converted to vitamin A (retinol) in the body. Only 50 per cent is absorbed and out of the absorbed only 50 per cent is converted to retinol.

It is essential for sound skin, tooth and bone health and development; it is also important in immune system function and the prevention of night blindness. Like vitamin C, it also plays the role of an antioxidant.

Major food sources of retinol are liver, fish oils, eggs, ghee, butter, milk and that of beta carotene are dark green leafy vegs, yellow and orange fruits and vegetables like carrots, papaya, mango and egg yolk. In an Indian diet, beta carotene provides most of the vitamin A necessary in human nutrition.

Vitamin A is lost from the food by deep-fat frying, by the use of defatted/low fat milk, oxidation and exposure to light. Malabsorption of fats, cholesterol-lowering drugs, and high fibre intake affect vit A absorption in the body.

Vitamin D

It is also known as the "sunshine vitamin". It is synthesised in the body by exposure to sunlight.

Two forms of vitamin D are important for nutrition:

- **Vitamin D_2 (ergocalciferol):** This form is synthesized from plants and yeast precursors. It is also the form used in very high dose supplements.
- **Vitamin D_3 (cholecalciferol):** This form is the most active form of vitamin D. It is formed in the skin when the skin is exposed to direct sunlight. The most common food source is fortified foods, mainly cereals and dairy products. Vitamin D_3 is also present in fish liver oils and

fatty fish. Cholecalciferol serves as a precursor to the hormonal form 1,25-dihydroxyvitamin D3 (calcitriol).

Vitamin D is stored mainly in the liver. Vitamins D_2 and D_3 are not active in the body. Both forms must be processed (metabolized) by the liver and kidneys into an active form called calcitriol. This active form promotes absorption of calcium and phosphorus from the intestine.

Functions:

1. Regulates the ***calcium and phosphorus*** levels in the blood by promoting their absorption from food in the intestines, and by promoting re-absorption of calcium in the kidneys.
2. It ***promotes bone formation*** and mineralization and is essential in the development of an intact and strong skeleton.
3. It ***inhibits parathyroid hormone*** secretion from the parathyroid gland.
4. Affects the ***immune system*** by promoting phagocytosis (The process by which a cell engulfs particles such as bacteria, other micro-organisms, aged red blood cells, foreign matter, etc.), anti-tumor activity, and immunomodulatory functions.

Sources: Endogenous production is the most important source. Vitamin D occurs naturally in animal foods. The richest source is fish liver oils like cod liver oil and small amounts are present in fatty fish, butter, cream, egg yolk and liver.

Deficiency: In vitamin D deficiency, calcium and phosphate levels in the blood decrease because vitamin D is necessary for absorption of these minerals. Because not enough calcium and phosphate are available to maintain healthy bones, vitamin D deficiency may result in a bone disorder called rickets in children or osteomalacia and osteoporosis in adults. Vitamin D deficiency makes osteoporosis worse. To try to increase the low calcium level in blood caused by vitamin D deficiency, the body may produce more parathyroid hormone. However, as the parathyroid hormone level becomes high (a condition called hyperparathyroidism), the hormone draws calcium out of bone to increase the calcium level in blood. Thus, the bones are weakened.

The most common cause is inadequate exposure to sunlight. Thus, vitamin D deficiency occurs mainly among people who do not spend much time outdoors.

Vitamin D and Diabetes

Study 1: Vitamin D deficiency predisposes individuals to Types 1 and 2 diabetes.

Vitamin D deficiency predisposes individuals to type 1 and type 2 diabetes, and receptors for its activated form—1α, 25-dihydroxyvitamin D3—have been identified in both beta cells and immune cells. Vitamin D deficiency has been shown to impair insulin synthesis and secretion in humans and in animal models of diabetes, suggesting a role in the development to type 2 diabetes.

Study 2: Vitamin D and Calcium Intake in Relation to Type 2 Diabetes in Women

Vitamin D deficiency is associated with insulin resistance and impaired pancreatic beta cell function. In this study it was found that both vitamin D and calcium intakes were inversely associated with development of type 2 diabetes, and the benefits of the two nutrients appeared to be additive. For both vitamin D and calcium, intakes from supplements rather than from diet were significantly associated with a lower risk of type 2 diabetes. Abnormal regulation of intracellular calcium affecting both insulin sensitivity and insulin release has been suggested as a potential mechanism to explain the association between calcium insufficiency and risk of diabetes.

Vitamin E

Vitamin E (tocopherol) is an antioxidant: It protects cells against damage by free radicals and also prevents oxidation of LDL cholesterol thus playing a role in prevention of CVD.

Its utilisation depends upon presence of dietary fat and it is lost by deep fat frying.

A very low fat diet lacks vitamin E because vegetable oils are the main source of this vitamin. Other sources of this vitamin are nuts, wheat germ, green leafy vegetables, eggs, liver and muscle meats. Disorders that impair fat absorption can also reduce the absorption of vitamin E and increase the risk of vitamin E deficiency.

Since dietary fats contain vit E, dietary deficiency is unlikely.

Vitamin K

Vitamin K has two forms:

- **Phylloquinone:** This form occurs in plants and is consumed in the diet. It is absorbed better when it is consumed with fat.
- **Menaquinone:** This form is produced by bacteria in the intestine, but only small amounts of it can be absorbed. In some countries, this form is used for supplementation.

Vitamin K is necessary for the synthesis of the proteins that help control bleeding (clotting factors) and thus for the normal clotting of blood. It is also needed for healthy bones and other tissues.

Sources include green lealfy vegetables (content proprotional to chlorophyll content), soya oil, cottonseed oil and olive oil.

MINERALS

Sodium

Most of the body's sodium is located in the blood and in the fluid in the space surrounding the cells (ECF). Sodium is required by all cells in the body to maintain a normal fluid balance. Sodium plays a key role in normal nerve and muscle function. It is taken in through food and drink and lost primarily in sweat and urine. Healthy kidneys maintain a consistent level of sodium in the body by adjusting the amount excreted in the urine.

Some important functions are as follows:

1. Maintains water balance (major electrolyte in ECF)
2. Maintains BP
3. Transmission of nerve impulses and muscle contractions
4. Transport of sugar and amino acids (Na/K/Ca ATPase pump).

Sources: Salt, bakery products, processed foods like cornflakes, pizzas, ajinomoto, cheese, salted butter, packet soups, pickles, papad, sauces and ketchups, namkeen like sev, chivda, farsaan, wafers, chips, salted nuts, salted popcorn, fast foods, cooking soda, baking soda (1 tsp = 1000 mg sodium), dried sea food, some drugs like some antacids and laxatives.

- Table salt is 40 per cent sodium;
  1 tsp of table salt = 2,400 mg of sodium.
- ADA recommends sodium intake of less than 2400 mg/day (i.e. 1 tsp of salt/day)

Hyponatremia

In hyponatremia, the level of sodium in the blood is too low (<135 meq/L). Hyponatremia occurs when sodium has been overdiluted in the body. Sodium can be overdiluted when people drink enormous amounts of water and as a result the amount of fluid taken in exceeds the kidneys' capacity to eliminate the excess. Other reasons could be diarrhoea, vomiting, burns, use of diuretics or extremely low intake.

Symptoms include loss of appetite, nausea, vomiting, headache, fatigue, irritability, lethargy, confusion, muscle twitching, seizures and coma.

Hypernatremia

In hypernatremia, the level of sodium in the blood is too high (>145 meq/l). The body contains too little water relative to the amount of sodium. The sodium level in the blood becomes abnormally high when water loss exceeds sodium loss, as occurs with dehydration. In most people, hypernatremia results from dehydration.

Hypernatremia occurs in people who drink too little water and in those who have diarrhoea, vomiting, fever, excessive sweating (particularly during hot weather), or abnormal kidney function. Symptoms include dizziness due to hypotension, vomiting, diarrhoea, edema.

Ways to Lower Sodium Intake:

1. Cook without added salt; use the prescribed amount of salt separately.
2. Add little or no salt at the table.
3. Read labels, looking for sodium content.
4. Choose fresh, frozen food items without added salts.
5. Select unsalted nuts.
6. Avoid salty snacks, like chips and namkeen.
7. Select unsalted soups or make them fresh at home.
8. Avoid junk foods, cooking soda, bakery products and processed foods.
9. Select fat-free or low-fat milk, low-sodium, low-fat cheeses, as well as low-fat curd.

10. Ask for your dish to be prepared without salt and/or ajinomoto when dining out.
11. Use spices and herbs to enhance the taste of your food; ex. Lime, tamarind, tomato, vinegar, ginger, garlic, mint.

Potassium

Most of the body's potassium is located inside the cells (ICF). Potassium is necessary for the normal functioning of cells, nerves, and muscles.

The level of potassium in the blood must be maintained within a narrow range. A potassium level that is too high or too low can have serious consequences, such as an abnormal heart rhythm or even cardiac arrest.

Kidney is the major excretory organ for potassium. Normal serum potassium = 3.5–5 meq/*l*.

Some important functions are as follows:

1. Maintains water balance
2. Nerve impulse transmission and muscle contraction
3. Regulation of BP.
4. Required for normal growth and muscle building.

Sources are green leafy vegetables, fruits like sweet lime, chiku, watermelon, mango, cherries, litchis, peach, fruit juices and vegetable soups, coconut water, fresh or dry coconut, pulses and legumes, potato with skin, milk and milk products.

Hypokalemia

In hypokalemia, the level of potassium in the blood is too low (<3.5 meq/l). Excessive potassium loss usually results from vomiting, diarrhoea and chronic laxative use. Very occasionally, excessive loss results from excessive sweating in conditions of extreme heat and humidity. Many foods contain potassium, so hypokalemia is rarely caused by too little intake in people who eat a balanced diet.

There are several reasons why potassium may be lost in the urine. By far the most common is the use of diuretics that cause the kidneys to excrete excess sodium, water, and potassium.

A mild decrease in the potassium level in the blood usually causes no symptoms. A more severe decrease can cause loss of appetite, mood changes, hypertension, loss of GI tone, elevated blood sugar, muscle weakness, twitches, and even paralysis. Abnormal heart rhythms may develop, especially in people with heart disease.

Hyperkalemia

In hyperkalemia, the level of potassium in the blood is too high. Hyperkalemia usually results when the kidneys do not excrete enough potassium. It can also result when a large amount of potassium is suddenly released from the cells. A sudden release of potassium from the cells can result from crush injuries (involving the destruction of large amounts of muscle tissue) and severe burns. The rapid movement of potassium from the cells into the bloodstream can overwhelm the kidneys and result in life-threatening hyperkalemia.

Other causes include GI bleed, severe infection, high intake of salt substitutes and use of potassium-sparing diuretics.

Symptoms include irregular heart beat (heart attack), nausea, slow/weak pulse.

Low potassium fruits include Guava, Apple, Pear, Papaya, Pineapple, Jamun, Orange, Banana (moderate)

Calcium

Most of the body's calcium is stored in the bones, but calcium is also found in cells (particularly muscle cells) and in the blood. Calcium is essential to muscle contraction and to the normal functioning of many enzymes. It is necessary for the formation of bone and teeth, for blood clotting, and for normal heart rhythm.

The body precisely controls the amount of calcium in the cells and the blood. Calcium content in the blood plasma is maintained within the narrow range of 9-11 mg/dl. Maintaining a normal level of calcium in the blood depends on consuming at least 1,000 to 1,500 milligrams of calcium a day and excreting excess calcium in urine. Calcium moves out of the bones into the bloodstream as needed to maintain a steady level of calcium in the blood. However, mobilizing too much calcium from the bones weakens them and can lead to osteoporosis.

Functions

1. Bone Formation: The important minerals within bone are calcium, phosphorus and magnesium.
2. Tooth Formation
3. Growth
4. Blood Clotting (Factor 4)
5. Regulates muscle contraction
6. Nerve impulse conduction
7. As a co-factor necessary for many enzyme reactions:

    a. Absorption of vitamin B12
    b. In the action of fat digesting enzyme, pancreatic lipase.
    c. In the **secretion of insulin from the pancreas**

Sources include dairy products (richest source), dark green leafy vegetables like colocassia (patra) leaves, cauliflower greens, amaranth leaves, cow pea (chawli) leaves, methi, lettuce, Ragi (nachni), legumes, almonds, black til, gardencress seeds, ravas, soybean and its products like tofu, soya milk.

Factors that enhance calcium absorption

1. Acid
2. Normal gastrointestinal motility
3. Phosphorus
4. Vitamin D
5. Need for calcium

6. Lactose
7. PTH

1. Acid

Calcium is more soluble and easily absorbed in acidic conditions.

2. GI motility

Normal motility of the GI favours calcium absorption.

3. Phosphorus

An increase in the amount of phosphate in the diet results in a reduction in the amount of calcium excreted. There is an inverse relationship between the dietary phosphorus intake and urinary calcium.

4. Vitamin D

The presence of the active form of vitamin D can result in a 10-30 per cent increase in dietary calcium absorption.

Low vitamin D intakes or inadequate exposure to sunlight reduce calcium absorption, especially among the elderly.

5. Need for calcium

During pregnancy, lactation and adolescence when calcium needs are greatest absorption efficiency is as high as 50 per cent.

Also, when calcium intakes are low, the body adapts by absorbing a greater proportion of the dietary calcium available and excreting less.

6. Lactose

The lactose in breast milk improves calcium absorption in human infants.

Beyond infancy it is doubtful whether lactose improves the absorbability of calcium from dairy products.

7. Parathyroid Hormone (PTH)

PTH helps maintain normal serum calcium.

Low serum calcium stimulates the release of PTH, which in turn promotes increased intestinal absorption of calcium *via* activated vitamin D.

Factors that hinder calcium absorption

1. Inadequate vitamin D intake
2. Alkaline conditions
3. Impaired GI motility
4. Imbalance in calcium phosphorus ratio
5. Phytic and oxalic acid
6. Excessive use of laxatives
7. Steatorrhea.
8. High fibre intake
9. Lack of exercise
10. Ageing
11. Caffeine
12. Drugs
13. Excessive sodium intake
14. High intake of zinc, iron or magnesium.
15. Excessive intake of alcohol
16. Smoking
17. Stress
18. Fat malabsorption

5. Phytates and Oxalates

Phytic acid present in cereals prevents calcium absorption by forming an insoluble complex with calcium.

Foods rich in phytates include whole grain cereals like bajra, jowar, whole wheat flour, ragi, pulses and legumes.

Fermentation, as occurs during bread making, reduces phytic acid because of the phytase present in yeast.

Oxalic acid present in spinach forms an insoluble complex with calcium (calcium-oxalate) which cannot be absorbed. Only 5 per cent of the calcium in spinach is absorbed.

Other foods containing oxalates are chocolate, cocoa, tea, amaranth, beer, juices containing berries (rasberry/strawberry), dried figs, whole wheat bread, wheat germ, roasted peanuts, til seeds.

6. *Excessive use of laxatives*

Laxatives increase the rate of passage of food through the intestinal tract this decreases calcium absorption by reducing the time available for the absorption to occur.

7. *Steatorrhea*

During steatorrhea (large foul smelling stools containing unabsorbed fat) calcium absorption is certainly reduced. This is because the malabsorbed fat forms insoluble soaps with calcium, preventing its absorption.

8. *High fibre intake*

Fibre reduces the absorption of calcium and other minerals by increasing the rate of passage of food through the intestinal tract. This decreases calcium absorption by reducing the time available for the absorption to occur. It also binds minerals within the structure thus making them unavailable for absorption. (only if > 30 g/d).

9. *Lack of exercise*

People who do not engage in weight-bearing exercises, such as walking, and bed-ridden people who are essentially immobile, can lose as much as 0.5 per cent of bone in a month and have a reduced ability to replace it. This may an important cause of calcium loss and decreased bone strength and mass in old people.

10. Ageing

Calcium absorption is decreased during old age. This may be due to lack/inadequate amount of hydrocholoric acid in the stomach and/or inadequate exposure to sunlight, increasing the risk of fractures.

11. Excessive sodium intake

Sodium and calcium excretion are linked in the proximal tubule of the kidney. Excess sodium can increase calcium excretion. Each gram of sodium leads to the urinary excretion of about 15 mg of calcium when calcium intake is high or moderate.

12. Caffeine

High intakes of caffeine affect the bio-availability of calcium by increasing the loss of calcium in urine. Daily consumption of the amount of caffeine in 3.5 cups of coffee or 7 cups of tea, has been shown to almost double the risk of developing osteoporosis.

13. Drugs

Some medications like anticoagulants, cortisone and thyroxine reduce calcium absorption as a side effect.

14. Excess intake of Fe, zinc or mg

They share the same absorption pathway with ca. Hence, excessive intakes of these minerals results in a competition between them for absorption.

15. Excessive alcohol intake

Drinking an average of 3 or more alcoholic drinks per day is clearly associated with an increased risk of osteoporosis. It has been well-established that even small doses of alcohol interfere with the absorption and use of both calcium and vitamin D.

16. Smoking

Greater incidence of osteoporosis was found among smokers than non-smokers.

17. Stress

Stress is also known to interfere with the body's ability to absorb minerals, including calcium.

18. Fat malabsorption

Calcium absorption is decreased because of the formation of calcium-fatty acid soaps.

RDA: 400 mg/d

Iron

There are two major pools of iron in the human body:

1. Functional Iron: Haemoglobin, myoglobin and enzymes.

2. Storage Iron: Ferritin, haemosiderin and transferrin.

Daily losses of iron are through GIT, skin, urine and menstrual blood losses.

Food contains two types of iron: heme iron (found in animal products) and non-heme iron (found in plant foods and in iron supplements). Non-heme iron accounts for more than 85 per cent of iron in the average diet. However, less than 20 per cent of non-heme iron that is consumed is absorbed into the body. Non-heme iron is absorbed better when it is consumed with animal protein and with vitamin C. Heme iron is absorbed much better than non-heme iron.

Functions:

1. Enables the transport of oxygen from lungs to the tissues.
2. Stores oxygen in muscle tissue.
3. Co-factor of many enzymes which carry out several vital functions in the body.

4. Essential for a healthy immune system and mental function.

Sources: Richest animal source is liver followed by oysters, seafoods, lean meat, poultry, egg yolk and fish. Plant sources include dark green leafy vegetables like amaranth, cauliflower greens, til seeds.

Iron Absorption From Indian Diets

- Adult men, children and adolescent boys—3 per cent
- Women, lactating women and adolescent girls—5 per cent
- Pregnant women—8 per cent

Factors increasing absorption are as follows:

1. Vitamin C
2. Acidic pH of the intestinal contents
3. Body need
4. Meat protein factor
5. Increased intestinal motility

1. Vitamin C

It is the most potent enhancer of iron absorption. It forms a chelate with iron that remains soluble at the alkaline pH of the lower small intestine. It enhances non-heme iron absorption especially well in women low iron intakes.

2. Acidic pH of the intestinal contents

It keeps iron in the soluble form and improves bio-availability.

3. Body's need

During pregnancy and growth, which demand increased blood formation, there is increased iron absorption. In iron-deficiency anemia also, more iron is absorbed.

4. Meat protein factor

Animal proteins from beef, pork, lamb, liver, fish and chicken enhance absorption. Substance responsible is known as the "Meat Protein Factor" (MPF). Mechanism unknown.

5. Increased intestinal motility

It decreases contact time. It rapidly removes the chyme from the area of highest intestinal acidity.

Factors that decrease absorption:

1. Phytates (*form insoluble complexes*)
2. Oxalates (*form insoluble complexes*)
3. Tannins
4. Dietary fibre (*increases transit time and acts as binder*)
5. Excess intake of zinc, manganese, calcium taken as supplements. (*absorption competition*)
6. Lack of stomach acid (*Makes non-heme iron insoluble*)
7. Antacids.

Iron Deficiency

Iron deficiency is the most common mineral deficiency in the world, causing anemia in men, women, and children.

In adults, iron deficiency is most commonly caused by loss of blood. In premenopausal women, monthly menstrual bleeding may cause the deficiency. Other causes are inadequate intake and malabsorption.

When iron reserves in the body are exhausted, anemia develops. Anemia causes paleness, weakness, irritability, drowsiness, and fatigue. Concentration and learning ability may be impaired. When severe, anemia may cause headache, ringing in the ears (tinnitus), spots before the eyes, digestive upset, shortness of breath, dizziness, and a rapid heart rate. Occasionally, severe anemia causes chest pain and heart failure. Menstrual periods may stop.

RDA: 30mg/d

Exchange List

Exchange	*Amount (g)*	*Calories (Kcal)*	*CHO (gms)*	*Protein (gms)*	*Fat (gms)*	*Fibre (mg)*
Cereal	30	100	21	2.5	0.5	0.6
Pulse	30	100	17	7	0.5	1.5
Cow's milk	100	70	4	3.2	4	—
Buffallo's milk	100	117	5	4.3	6.5	—
Mutton	50	100	—	8	7	—
Egg	1 no.	85	—	6.5	6.5	—
Fish or chicken	100	100	—	20.0	2.0	—
Vegetable A	100	25	6	1.0	—	1.2
Vegetable B	100	50	10	1.0	0.5	0.8
Vegetable C	100	100	24	1.0	—	0.7
Fruit	100	50	10	—	—	1.75
Soyabean	20	90	4	9	4	0.7
Sugar	5	20	5	—	—	—
Fat (1 tsp)	5	45	—	—	5	—
Coconut (dry)	15	100	2.5	1.02	10	0.9
Coconut (fresh)	25	100	3.0	1.12	10.4	0.9
Groundnut	15	100	8.0	3.79	6.0	0.5
Marie biscuit	4 no.	60				
Glucose biscuit	3 no.	110				

Edible Portions of Coconut

Coconut (Edible Portion)	*Fresh*	*Dry*
Small	175 g	—
Big	250 g	—
Standard	—	80 g.

Fruit Exchanges for Diabetic Patients

All fruits in the exchange list provide 10g CHO

Apple	1 small/½ medium
Guava	1 medium
Orange	1 medium
Papaya	1/3 medium or 3 slices}= 12-14 pc"cube
Pineapple	2-3 slices
Pear	1 medium
Sweet lime	1 medium
Watermelon	2-3 slices
Pomegranate	1/3rd medium
Coconut water	150 ml
Jamun	100 gm
High Calorie Fruits	
Banana	½ big
Mango	½ medium (75 g)
Chickoo	1 small
Sitaphal	(50g) ½ big size
Grapes	12-15 pieces

Thumb Rules for Making a Diet Plan

- **Time**
  Minimum 3 hrs gap between two major meals
- **Cereals**
  Rule:

No. of Cereal Exchanges

Actual	1-2	>2-<4	>,=4
Read Reduction	0	1	2

  √ Total cereal exchanges not < 6/day
  √ Balance each meal
  √ Potato = cereal
- **PULSES**
  √ 2.5 exchanges of pulses/day (including soya)
  √ Min of 1 exchange each in lunch and dinner

√ Max 1 exchange/d can be replaced 2-3 times/wk with:
√ Low fat paneer—1 med k *OR*
√ Egg whites—2 no. *OR*
√ Fish/Chicken-2 pieces.

- **FRUITS**
  √ Permitted no. of fruit exchanges/day = 2
  √ Food and fruit gap to be 2 hours.
- **FAT**
  √ Visible fat allowance = 3-5 t/d (15-25 g/d)
- **SUGAR, JAGGERY AND HONEY**
  √ Completely avoid.
- **MILK AND PRODUCTS**
  √ Convert to low fat versions like toned/double toned/ skimmed cow milk/skim milk.
  √ Even paneer and curds to be made from the same low fat milk.
- **NON-VEG**
  √ Egg whites, fish and chicken acceptable
  √ Grilled, roasted, boiled, onion-tomato gravy-mode of cooking.
  √ Red meat to be completely avoided
- **NUTS AND OILSEEDS**
  √ Stop coconut (fresh, dry and milk), til and groundnut intake completely.
- **ALCOHOL**
  √ Advice to stop
  √ Reduce frequency and quantity by half
- **MISCELLANEOUS**
  √ No bed-time snacks
  √ Pre-exercise/walk: 1 cup milk/coffee, 1 excahnge fruit, 1 fistful kurmura-channa
  √ Mid-meal snacks to be protein-rich
  √ Salt allowance—1 levelled teaspoon/day.
  √ Avoid/Replace junk food with healthier options
  √ Follow Dr's advice regarding timing of medicine consumption.

Nutrition Therapy for Diabetes

Diabetes mellitus is a chronic disease, without a cure, and emphasis must necessarily be on managing/avoiding possible short-term as well as long-term diabetes-related problems. There is an exceptionally important role for patient education, dietetic support, regular exercise, self-glucose monitoring with the goal of keeping both short-term blood glucose levels and long-term levels as well, within acceptable bounds.

Management of diabetes involves 5 important pillars. These include:

1. **Medication**—It includes both oral medicines and insulin depending on the patient's type and levels of blood glucose of diabetes. It is extremely important to follow the doctor's advice for the same.
2. **Medical Nutrition Therapy**—Medical Nutrition Therapy (MNT) is a medically necessary and cost effective way of treating and controlling many diseases and medical conditions. It involves the assessment of nutritional status followed by therapy. It is integral to total diabetes care and management.
3. **Exercise**—Exercise can be defined as physical activity that is a planned, structured movement of the body designed to enhance physical fitness.
4. **Monitoring**—A way of testing how much glucose (sugar) is in the blood. It can be done at the lab and also at home using a device called glucometer. The process of monitoring blood sugars at home is known as Self-Monitoring of Blood Glucose (SMBG).

SMBG can aid in diabetes control by:

- facilitating the development of an individualized blood glucose profile, which can then guide health care professionals in treatment planning for an individualized diabetic regimen;

- giving people with diabetes and their families the ability to make appropriate day-to-day treatment choices in diet and physical activity as well as in insulin or other agents;
- improving patients' recognition of hypoglycemia or severe hyperglycemia;
- enhancing patient education and patient empowerment regarding the effects of lifestyle and pharmaceutical intervention on glycemic control.

5. **Lifestyle**—It involves a person's pattern of living as expressed by their interests, motivations, activities, desired experiences, and beliefs. For e.g. intake of alcohol and smoking is one of the components of lifestyle and affects the blood sugars. Therefore, lifestyle management is also one of the important pillars for managing diabetes.

Role of MNT in diabetes: MNT like in any other condition performs the following role:

a. Encompasses clinical principles—it includes the guidelines that are to be followed. For e.g. 1 g protein/kg present wt.
b. Individual circumstances—it means that MNT takes into individual circumstances not by applying the same norms to everyone as each one of us is different.
c. Cultural and ethnic preferences—likewise our circumstances, there is a variation in cultural and ethnic backgrounds. Therefore, MNT is flexible.
d. Maintains lifestyle changes—as discussed earlier lifestyle modification has an important role to play in DM management. Therefore it is an integral part of MNT.

Goals of MNT for Diabetes

- To attain and maintain optimal metabolic outcomes including

— Blood glucose levels in the normal range.
— Lipid and lipoprotein profile that reduces the risk for vascular disease—levels of LDL, HDL, TG within the range.
— Blood pressure levels in the normal range or as close to normal as is safely possible.

- To prevent, or at least slow, the rate of development of chronic complications of diabetes—nutrient and lifestyle modification.
- To address individual nutritional needs, taking into consideration personal, cultural preferences and lifestyle.
- To maintain the pleasure of eating by only limiting food choices when indicated by scientific evidence.—entire diet of the patient should not be changed. The modifications made should hold a scientific basis. For e.g. a patient has total Cholesterol—300mg/dl and his consumption of saturated fats is high. Therefore, his intake of SFAs needs to be restricted.

Insulin secretagogues are medicines that work by making the body produce more insulin from the pancreas. (Insulin is the hormone that normally controls blood glucose levels). These are meal dependent medicines (may lead to hypoglycemia if meals are delayed or skipped) and should be taken as prescribed with the balance in diet.

This brings us to answer a question, ***is there any diabetic diet?*** There is no diet called as diabetic diet. The plan advised should be ***Nutritionally adequate*** i.e. it should meet with all the requirements of nutrients of the individual; ***Individualized*** i.e. we cannot have one plan for suiting and meeting every patient's requirement and targets; ***Flexible*** i.e. the plan should give options in diet (during travel or eat out or socializing) and ensure that the patient gets choices and variety maintaining his/her requirements for achieving their glycemic goal.

Key steps for an ideal diet plan

Following steps may help constructing a diet plan:

- **Assess the patients medical history, BMI, physical activity and diet history**

  Medical history means "A list of a person's previous illnesses, present conditions, symptoms, medicines, and health risk factors."

  BMI is a measure of the relative body fatness to evaluate risk factors associated with obesity. It is based on weight (in kg) with minimal clothing and height (in metres) without shoes.

Grade	BMI (kg/m^2)
Under weight	< 18.5
Normal	18.5-22.9
Grade 1	23-24.9
Grade 2	25-29.9
Grade 3	>= 30

  Physical activity can be classified in various forms as sedentary, Moderate, active, bed ridden.

  Diet history is a method of dietary assessment in which subjects are asked to recall their food consumption over a specific period of time. ***Diet recall***

  Assessment = Medical History + Physical Activity Level + Diet History

  Nutrition assessment is used to determine what the individual with diabetes is able and willing to do

- **Determine caloric requirements**

Obese	20 Kcal/kg
Sedentary, inactive (men/women) Between 35yrs-55yrs	22-25 Kcal/kg
Sedentary (men/women) 55 yrs and above	28 Kcal/kg
(sedentary men/active women) Active (men/women)	30 Kcal/kg
Thin/Very active, Men	40 Kcal/kg

***Points to remember*:** Calories and protein prescribed should be based on present weight.

Strategies may be aimed at improving food selection (e.g. reducing fats and saturated fats), spreading meals throughout the day, and regular exercise.

- **Determine dietary distribution of proximal principles Carbohydrates, CHO_4, Protein, Fat.**
  The distribution of macro nutrients is based on patient's current eating pattern but with a focus on dietary norms to be applied.

Quick Guide on T2DM Diet Major/Macro Nutrients

CHO_4		*Protein*		*Fats*	
Simple Easily absorbed in blood	*Complex Gradual absorption in blood*	*Class 1 Good quality*	*Class 2 Moderate quality*	*Visible Added while cooking*	*Invisible Present before cooking*
Sugar	Roti	Toned milk	All Dals	Refined Oil	Fish
Jam	Dalia	Egg white	Cereals	(all kinds)	Chicken
Honey	Restricted Oats	Paneer		Desi ghee	Mutton
Mithai	Whole	Curds		Processed	Eggs
Biscuit	Wheat	Fish		Cheese	Milk
Soft drinks	Bread	Chicken		Dalda	Nuts
Fruit juice	Raw fruits	Soybean		Margarine	Dals
White Bread	Vegetables	*Daily protein = 1 g/kg*		Cream/	Cereals
Plain Rice		*present wt If nephropathy*		Malai	
Poha	*Moderate*	= 0.8-1.0g/kg* If obese		*Daily visible fat intake-*	
Suji	*amounts*	*= 1g/kg ideals body wt*		3tsp-5tsp/day*	
Idli		*50% daily protein from*		* there could be individual	
Dosa		*CLASS I sources*		*variation*	
50% total calories from		*If veg pt, may recommend;*			
complex carbs		*Dals + Roti/Rice*			
		Milk(paneer/curds) + Rice/			
		Roti			

- **Formulation of meal plan.**
  After assessment and diet history it is the meal plan that needs to be planned as per the individual
- **Distribution of carbohydrates and calories in relation to physical activity and oral hypoglycemic agents throughout the day.**

***Sweeteners*:** Sweeteners are ingredients that add sweetness to foods like soft drinks, desserts, candies, pastries. There are 2 categories of sweetners.

a. Nutritive sweeteners—which have calories
b. Non-Nutritive sweeteners—

Nutritive Sweeteners

Sugar Name	*Description*
Sucrose	This form of carbohydrate is found in table sugar, raw sugar, cane sugar, powdered sugar and brown sugar. Sucrose is 50 per cent glucose and 50 per cent fructose.
Dextrose	Another name for glucose.
Honey	Honey is 35 per cent glucose and 40 per cent fructose, a close relative to Honey sucrose.
High Fructose Corn Syrup	Less expensive and sweeter than sucrose, it is primarily glucose. It is usually found in sodas and soft drinks.
Corn Syrup or Corn Sugar	Derived from cornstarch, this sugar is high in glucose.
Fructose	Fructose sweetener, fruit sugar. Because fructose is sweeter than sucrose, less can be used in recipes.
Maltose	Found in malt, beer. It is potent and adds quickly to the blood glucose pool. This is formed from 2 glucose molecules.

Another form of nutritive sweeteners include **Sugar alcohols.** They are:

- CHO with chemical structure that partially resembles both sugar and alcohol.

- Readily converts to sugar in liver, may also cause high TGs and wt gain.
- If taken in excess, may cause diarrhoea.
- 1g = 2 Kcal approx.

Sugar Name	*Description*
Sorbitol	Derived from glucose; this sweetener is 60 per cent as sweet as sucrose.
Xylitol	Derived from xylose, it is equal in sweetener to sucrose.
Isomalt	Derived from sucrose; it is about 60 per cent as sweet as sucrose.
Mannitol	Derived from mannose; it is about 70 per cent as sweet as sucrose.
Hydrogenated Starch Hydrolysates (HSH)	Derived from corn, wheat or potato starches. These sweeteners range from 40 per cent to 90 per cent as sweet as sucrose.

***Non-nutritive Sweeteners*:** Non-nutritive sweeteners are added in very small amounts to foods for a significant sweetening effect. These sweeteners have been approved for use in a number of dietetic or reduced-calorie foods and beverages. While safety is a concern, only minute amounts are necessary.

Saccharin	Saccharin is about 300 times as sweet as sucrose. It has been in use since the late 1800s and is a popular tabletop sweetener. In the 1970's, its safety was questioned in the United States because of studies suggesting an increased risk of bladder cancer in male rats given very high levels of saccharin. Later, the research design was called into question and its conclusions refuted. It is now determined that up to 1 gram per day of saccharin poses no health risks to adults. While there is no evidence of harmful effects reported, recent studies show that saccharin does cross the placenta and may be of concern to some women during pregnancy.

Acesulfame K	Acesulfame Potassium (K) is 200 times as sweet as sucrose. It is heat-stable so, unlike aspartame, it can be used in cooking. It is added to dry mixes for sugar free gelatins, puddings and beverages. It can also be used in baked goods. In Canada and Europe it is approved for soft drinks. There are no safety concerns raised about Acesulfame K. It has been deemed safe for all age groups.
Aspartame	Aspartame is 200 times sweeter than sucrose. It became available as a tabletop sweetener in the 1970s and is now added to thousands of foods. It is not stable in heat nor for long periods is liquid form. While the U.S. Food and Drug Administration stated that high heat or long storage times could decrease the quality of the food products, they concluded that this did not pose a health risk. The FDA has approved aspartame for use during pregnancy and lactation. The Centre for Disease Control did state that some individuals might be unusually sensitive to aspartame. Anyone who experiences a reaction to aspartame is encouraged to document it and discuss it with his or her physician. Phenylalanine is a component of aspartame that should be avoided by individuals with a rare metabolic disorder called phenylketonuria (PKU). Phenylalanine does cross the placenta and has been a concern in producing PKU in offspring. However, even at high levels of intake placental transport of this substances does not appear to be clinically harmful.
Sucralose	Sucralose is a non-caloric sweetener that is made from sugar. It was approved in April of 1998 for use as a table top sweetener. It is now used to sweeten products in more than 30 countries. Sucralose is 600 times sweeter than sugar and it is heat-stable, which means it can be used for baked goods. Sucralose has no effect on blood sugar, offers no calories and is deemed safe for use with all populations, including pregnant and lactating women as well as children.

Sweeteners	**Acceptable Dietary intake mgm/kgm body wt.**
ACESULFAME K (Sunette, Sweet One)	15 mg/kg body wt./day
ASPARTAME (Equal, Sugar free, Nutra Sweet)	50 mg/kg body wt./day
SACCHARIN	5 mg/kg body wt./day
SUCRALOSE (Splenda, Zero, Elata)	15 mg/kg body wt./day

***Micro-nutrients*:** When dietary intake is adequate, there is generally no need for additional vitamin and mineral supplementation for the majority of people with diabetes. Micro-nutrient should be supplemented/modified on indication. Restircted diets usually require supplementation.

***Hypoglycemia*:** is low blood sugar. When blood sugars fall below <70mg/dl, it is diagnosed as hypoglycemia in a diabetes patient.

Changes in food intake, physical activity, medication(s) except JANUVIA can contribute to the development of hypoglycemia.

- Glucose is the preferred treatment for hypoglycemia,
- Ingestion of 15-20 g of glucose is effective.

***Hypertension*:** A reduction in sodium intake lowers BP. Goal should be to reduce Na intake to 1 tsf/day (levelled). Modest amount of weight loss beneficially affects BP.

***Diabetes Nephropathy*:** Nephropathy means kidney disease or damage. Diabetic nephropathy is damage to your kidneys caused by diabetes. In severe cases it can lead to kidney failure.

The kidneys have many tiny blood vessels that filter waste, electrolytes (sodium, potassium and phosphorus) and water from your blood. High blood sugar from diabetes can destroy these blood vessels. Over time, the kidney isn't able to do its job as well. Later it may stop working completely. This is called kidney failure.

Dietary Management of diabetes nephropathy

- Work with your doctor to keep your blood pressure in the target range.
- Keep your heart healthy by eating a low-fat diet and exercising regularly.

- Watch how much protein you eat. Eating too much is hard on your kidneys. Reduction of dietary protein of 0.8-1.0g/kg/day and for people with micro albuminuria a reduction to 0.8 g/kg/day.
- Keep a check on your salt intake and overall sodium in the diet.
- Don't smoke or use other tobacco products.

Disadvantages of Over Cooking

Lately lot of attention has been diverted to the harmful effects of various methods of cooking. *It was earlier felt that over cooking kills bacteria and makes the food sterile and safe for eating and therefore a lot of people had erred on the side of over cooking rather than under cooking. It certainly helps in killing bacteria but recent research has shown a lot of harmful effects of over cooking.*

1. It has been shown that by *over cooking or exposing food to high temperature for long periods of time, sugars get converted into Advanced Glycation End products (AGE's) which irritate the cells of the body and release certain triggers of inflammation like C Reactive Protein.* These advanced glycation end products are associated with disorders *commonly found* in adults as they get older *like hypertension* (High Blood Pressure), *diabetes, stroke, dementia, vision problems, skin changes,* nervous system and skin disorders. *AGE's* are produced more with *animal derived products,* for example *cheese, bacon and sausages* on exposure to *high temperature.* If one adds water, specially the use of *steaming,* it delays *this* reaction leading to the *production of AGE's* and is therefore beneficial. *Dry high temperature* is the worst *culprit* in this matter.
2. It has been shown that exposure of starch rich food (*such as fried potatoes, potato chips, some* types of *breakfast careals and baked food*) *to high* temperature *leads to production* of *a substance* called "*Acrylamide*" which is a *cancer producing* substance and has been associated with some forms of cancer. This fact has been borne out

of research carried out in the University of Stockholm. Heating the amino acid "Asparagine" with sugars at temperatures upwards of 120 degree centigrade causes production of Acrylamides. *Frying, baking,* roasting and *grilling for long periods* are *most* likely to reach these *temperatures* and may be *harmful.* Even use of *pasteurised food especially* milk may be harmful.

3. Also certain vitamins, specially *water soluble Vitamins B, C and E,* are *dramatically unstable* and they get *destroyed on exposure to* high temperature.
4. Over cooking also *reduces the carotene level* of the *food and therefore Vitamin A (which is very* important for proper vision and *for development* of retina), gets *depleted* in the food.
5. Repeated exposure to high temperature, specially *repeated frying of vegetables, Samosas and Pakoras in the same oil again and again,* leads to production of a special form *of fat called "Trans Fatty Acids", which are extremely dangerous as they deposit in the wall of the arteries leading to their clogging and blocking.* Depending on the area or the organ of the body where these trans fatty acids lodge *are the* effects *noticed.* For example if trans fatty acids get deposited in the arteries of the *heart, one can get heart attacks;* if in the arteries of *the brain,* one *gets stroke; in the eyes, it can lead to blindness*; in the *kidneys* to kidney *failure and in the legs* to *pain in the legs* on walking (*claudication*) and some *times even to gangrene ending ultimately with amputations.* These trans fatty acids are actually the atherogenic i.e. cholesterol depositing form of fat and are very *dangerous.*
6. Besides that over cooking leads to vegetables loosing their normal lustre so that they become dull and they also loose their delecate flavour and aroma of herbs which are very important for normal salivation and for digestion of food.

With so many disadvantages of *over cooking food, it* is *therefore just appropriate to know what is the best* cooking *method for good health of the* whole family. For a healthy heart, we must *eat food prepared* by such a cooking method that there is minimum loss of *nutrients*. There are various methods recommended for cooking:

a. ***Boiling*** **:** The simplest method of cooking is boiling. It is the cooking of *food in a* rapidly boiling liquid *at a temperature* of 100°C. But the main disadvantages being loss of *nutrients,* colour and flavour.
b. **Simmering :** When foods are cooked in a pan with a well *fitting lid* at a temperature just below the boiling point of the liquid in which they are immersed (water—82-99°C), the process is known as simmering. Advantage of this method is that loss of *nutrients* is less.
c. **Steaming :** To *retain the nutritive value of food, steaming is a very good method.* Steaming is the process of *cooking food in steam from a boiling* liquid, *usually water.* There is less loss of nutrients as there is no leaching *and* cooking time is less. Colour and flavour of vegetables is retained *in this* method.
d. **Pressure Cooking :** In pressure cooking, escaping steam is trapped and kept under pressure so that the temperature of the boiling water and steam can be raised *above 100°C* and reduce the cooking time. There is loss *of flavour* and colour.
e. **Grilling :** Cooking is done *under a source* of radient heat. There *is less loss of nutrients* and improved *flavour of food,* but one can do over cooking unless *one is* careful.
f. **Roasting :** When food is cooked uncovered on *heated metal* or frying *pan the method is known* as *roasting.* There is loss of nutrients *like* amino acids when the food becomes brown.
g. **Sautéing :** This method involves cooking in just enough of oil to cover the base of pan (greasing the pan). The heat is transformed to food mainly by conduction.

In general, *Frying, Grilling and Microwave cooking for long periods lead to very high temperatures as compared to boiling and steaming.* The ideal method of cooking, which is recommended, is *a combination of steaming and sautéing.*

The advantages which are seen by using these methods are:

a. Nutritive value of food is maintained because there is no leaching and cooking time is less.

b. Easily digestible and not much fat is added.

c. Texture of food is better, light and fluffy.

d. Flavour of sauted and steamed food is good.

e. It is ideal for those with poor digestion.

Diet for Specific Diseases

Diet in heart diseases

- Low Calorie, low fat, normal protein and high fibre diet should be taken.
- Restrict total calories to reduce body weight and to maintain it at ideal weight.
- Fat should not be more than 25-30 per cent of total calories intake.
- Saturated fats, hydrogenated vegetable oils, margarine, butter, ghee should be avoided.
- Fried foods like puri, paratha, mathi, namkeens, etc. should be avoided. Instead roasted namkeens and steamed food such as idli, dhokla etc. should be preferred.
- Rice bran oil, soybean oil, sunflower oil, olive oil, and mustard oil can be used. Blends of oil are preferred or change the oil every month.
- Fish oil is a good source of omega-3 fatty acids. Consumption of 100-200gm fish twice a week helps to lower down the cholesterol.
- Small meals should be taken instead of large meals.
- Skimmed milk and its milk products, cottage cheese should be taken. Avoid whole milk and its product—cream, khoya, etc.
- Red meat, organ meat, egg yolk should be avoided. Lean meat, fish, egg white can be taken.
- Avoid refined cereals, sugar starches, etc. prefer complex carbohydrates like whole-wheat flour, dalia, oatmeal, brown breads, bran biscuit etc.

- Commercial baked products like pies, cakes, biscuits, high fat crackers, and chocolates should be avoided.
- Antioxidants should be increased in the diet so three servings of vegetables and two servings of fruit should be given. Apples, oranges, guavas, pomegranate (anar), papaya, berries, pineapple, tomato, amla, onion are good sources of antioxidants.
- Fenugreek seeds, garlic, oat bran, bengal gram helps in reducing cholesterol level so they should be included in diet.
- Regular exercise should be done but physical strain after meal should be avoided.
- Smoking should be totally stopped and alcohol should be stopped or minimized.

Diet in Hypertension

- A low calorie, low fat, low sodium diet with normal protein intake should be taken.
- Maintain the weight near to your ideal body weight. If more, restrict your calorie intake to 1200-1500 kcal.
- Avoid animal fats, hydrogenated vegetable oils, margarine, butter, ghee, cream etc.
- A diet of 60 gm protein is necessary to maintain proper nutrition. Lean meat, fish, skimmed milk, cottage cheese, egg white; soybean should be included in the diet.
- Restricted sodium and decrease in sodium/potassium ratio in diet is preferred.
- Restrict the salt used in cooking. Low sodium salt can also be used.
- Avoid table salt and, salt preserved foods like pickles etc.
- Chutney, sauces, papad should be avoided.
- Highly salted foods like potato chips, namkeens, chaat etc. should be avoided.
- Canned and processed food, shellfish and dry fish, nuts, should be avoided.
- Bakery products prepared mixes should be avoided.
- Radish (muli), beetroot, carrot, peas, methi, palak, saag, lotus stem, tomato, lemon should be taken in restriction (once a weak).
- Fruit juices, aerated drinks, squashes, Jal-jeera, coconut water should be avoided.
- A high fibre diet should be taken. Include salads in every meal. Whole wheat flour, wheat breads, oatmeal, should be used instead of refined cereals.
- Follow a regular exercise plan.

Diet in Kidney Diseases

- Restrict the protein intake to the advised level.
- Avoid extra milk, fish, chicken, dals, legumes etc.
- Prefer giving proteins from high biological value protein sources like egg, lean meat, milk etc
- Rice is preferred to chapatti as they contain less protein.
- To reduce the potassium content soak the vegetables in water for 1-2 hrs and then drain out the water.
- If oedema is present then water intake should be less as advised.

Foods to be avoided are

- Legumes and pulses.
- Fried foods like paratha, samosa, pakora etc.
- Dry fruits like peanuts, cashew nuts, coconut, raisins (kishmish), khajur etc.
- Fruit juices, colas, squashes, sherbets etc.
- Alcohol and beer.
- Egg yolk, seafood, organ meat, cream cheese, ghee etc.
- Fruits like mango, banana, litchi, cheeku, grapes, musk-melon, lemon, mausami, apricots.
- Vegetable like arbi, jimikand, ganth gobi, lotus stem, green leafy vegetables like palak, methi, saag, radish, carrot (once a week).
- Salt preserved fish and meat.
- Canned and processed foods.
- No table salt, baking soda, ajinomoto
- Pulses like Bengal gram, lentil.

Diet to Avoid Hypoglycemia

- Eat small meals, with snacks interspersed between meals and at bedtime. This means having 5-6 meals rather 2-3 meals to steady the release of glucose into blood stream.
- Spread intake of carbohydrate throughout the day. Eat 2-4 servings of carbohydrate foods at each meal and 1-2 servings at each snack.
- Avoid excess use of beverages and food containing caffeine as it can cause the same symptoms as hypoglycemia and makes the individual feel worse.
- Limit or avoid alcoholic beverages. Drinking alcohol empty stomach and without food can lower glucose levels. Alcohol (if taken) should be in moderation (1-2 drinks no more than twice a week).
- Decrease fat intake. A high fat diet, especially saturated fats, has been shown to affect the body's ability to use insulin (insulin resistance).

Treatment of hypoglycemia

If blood glucose level falls below 70mg/dl immediately give carbohydrate rich food equivalent to 15 gm of carbohydrate (3 glucose biscuits, 1 table spoon ful of sugar, half cup fruit juice or softdrink). Wait for 15 minutes and retest, if sugar level remains less than 70 mg/dl give 15 gms more carbohydrate. Repeat until blood glucose level returns to normal.

Diet in Fever

- A high calorie, high protein, and soft diet is recommended.
- Selection of food should be from those bland in flavours, non-stimulating, less spicy and easily digested.
- Food should be appetizing and patients likes and dislikes should be considered.
- Initially small quantities of fluid diet should be given once in two-three hours. When fever comes down gradually normal food can be given.
- Giving good quality protein like eggs, milk, lean meat, soybean etc. to increase protein intake.
- Mixture of protein and carbohydrate is preferred.
- Fatty foods, spicy foods, highly fibrous foods that are hard to digest should be avoided.
- During diarrhoea and vomiting, ample amount of liquid should be consumed like small sips after every 15-30 min.

Foods to be included

Fruit juices, coconut water, barley water, milk and milk shakes (if there is no diarrhoea) custards, thin dals, curries, eggs, baked fish, cottage cheese, porridges, steamed vegetables juices, soups, etc.

Foods to be avoided

Butter, ghee, chillies and other spices, sugar rich pastries, fried foods, puddings, cream soups etc.

Dental Care in Diabetes

The most common major oral complication of diabetes is gum disease. If untreated, gum disease can be very serious and lead to tooth loss. To avoid if following things should be followed:

- Brush your teeth after every meal and before bedtime.
- Use fluoride toothpaste.
- Eat well balanced diet.
- Avoid foods high in sugar especially foods that stick to teeth like candies, caramels, raising etc.
- Visit to dental clinic every 3 months for cleaning, inspection, and oral hygiene instructions.

Diet during Dental Problems

A soft diet should be given. Dal and rice, dalia, khichdi, upma, poha, steamed or boiled vegetables, soups, porridges, unsweetened milk, etc. should be given which is not hard to chew. Increasing the steamed vegetables can increase fibre intake, oat bran or wheat bran can be mixed in soups etc.

Diabetes and Pregnancy

During pregnancy, glycosuria is not uncommon, because of the increased circulating blood volume and its load of metabolites. Most of these women revert to normal glucose tolerance after delivery, but have a greater likelihood of developing diabetes in later life, particularly if there is associated obesity.

Adjustment of insulin dosage in women with gestational diabetes, based on the results of post prandial rather than pre-prandial blood glucose values, improves glycemic control and decreases the risk of neonatal hypoglycemia, macrosomia, and caesarean delivery.

Ketosis in the mother causes intrauterine death or foetus deformity. Good diabetes control is therefore indispensable during pregnancy. It reduces the risk of toxemia, intrauterine death, macrosomia and neonatal hypoglycemia.

Diet Modifications for Diabetic Pregnant Women

1. From 3-6 months increased energy allowance is necessary for the mother for blood expansion and growth of uterus, breasts and fat stores while in last month, it is for growth of foetus and placenta.
2. 25-30 gms. of additional protein per day is recommended for mother daily. Daily supplement of 2-3 cups of milk and its product and one average helping of non-veg (fish, chicken, egg) or paneer, soybean is advised.
3. Supplement of multi-vitamin, iron, calcium, folic acid should be taken.
4. Regular exercise should be done.

5. Some suggested recipies during Pregnancy

	Reason
Dairy products like milk curd, yoghurt, cheese, paneer	To meet requirements of protein and calcium and vitamin D
Green leafy vegetables, whole grains, salads	Natural laxatives and prevent constipation
Fruit Salad	Appetising and provide many nutrients and fibre
Omlette, egg, chicken, fish	Good quality of protein and iron
Rice flakes, upma, puffed rice ball	Good source of iron and easy to digest
Pickles, rasam, sour foods	Give relief from nausea.

6. Diet should be high in fibre.
7. Avoid simple starches, sugar, honey, juices etc. which can increase blood sugar levels.
8. Small frequent meals should be taken.
9. Check the blood glucose level daily.

Diet for Liver Diseases

Diet for diabetic patient suffering from liver cirrhosis (1400kcal)

Milk	:	500 ml.
Egg/Paneer	:	60 gm.
Pulse	:	50 gm.
Wheat flour	:	80 gm.
Rice/Sago	:	100 gm.
Fruit	:	200 gm.
Vegetable	:	400 gm.
Fat	:	10 gm.

- High protein diet should be given in initial stage but if patient is in precoma or coma, protein should be withheld.
- If there is cirrhotic ascites (accumulation of fluid in abdominal area) then sodium intake is restricted.
- Bakery products, dried fruits, nuts, cream, spices, papad, chutney should be avoided.
- Green leafy vegetables radish, carrot etc. should be avoided.
- Fried preparation, whole milk, cream should be avoided.
- Medium chain triglycerides like coconut oil, olive oil is preferred.
- Alcoholic beverages should be strictly avoided.
- Animal protein like egg, meat should be restricted if there is increased blood ammonia.
- Protein from plant origin should be preferred.
- Combination of protein and cereal is preferred like porridge, puddings khichdi etc.

Food That Helps!

Garlic

Garlic is in the special food for discussion in this issue. We celebrate the unique flavour of garlic. It is guaranteed to transform any meal into a bold, aromatic and healthy culinary experience. Garlic is an indispensable addition to almost all cuisines throughout the world. Not only does it add bold and interesting flavour to your favourite savory recipe, it also provides a wealth of health-promoting benefits, such as reducing the risk of heart disease, lowering cholesterol levels and balancing blood sugar levels. So include a little garlic in your meal as a great way to add extra flavour and nutrition of your Healthiest Way of Eating!

Nutritional Value

One ounce of garlic (about 3 medium cloves) provides 24 per cent of the Daily Value (DV) for manganese, 18 per cent DV for vitamin B6, 15 per cent DV for vitamin C. Garlic's special sulfur compounds also provide powerful antioxidant protection against free radical damage to cellular structures, including DNA.

Health Benefits of GARLIC

Both the leaves and the roots of Garlic have been the subject of fascinating health studies. The combination of traditional nutrients, phytonutrients (particularly *anthocyans*) plus fibre in this food seems particularly effective in preventing digestive tract cancers.

If vegetables got grades for traditional nutrients alone, garlic would be one of the vegetable valedictorians. The vitamin and mineral profile of this leafy green vegetable contains enough "excellents" to ensure its place at the head of the vegetable Dean's List. The rating system awards garlic with excellent marks for its concentrations of vitamin K, vitamin A, vitamin C, magnesium, manganese, potassium, iron, vitamin E, and dietary fibre. It also emerges as a very good source of copper, calcium, vitamin B2, vitamin B6, protein, phosphorus, vitamin B1, zinc, folate, biotin, niacin and pantothenic acid.

Helping You Bone Up.

Garlic Gets an A+ for its Pro-vitamin A

Promotes Lung Health.

A Healthy Dose of Vitamin C for Antioxidant Protection and Immune Support.

Protects Your Heart with Potassium.

Iron for Energy.

Anti-Inflammatory and Cardiovascular Benefits.

An Excellent Source of Fibre.

Manganese-Energy Production Plus Antioxidant Protection.

Cardiovascular Protection Brought to You By Swiss Chard's Riboflavin and B6.

Vitamin E-rich Leafy Greens Slow Loss of Mental Function.

Eat to Live

What is the Glycemic Index?

Not all carbohydrate foods (carbs) are created equal, in fact they behave quite differently in our bodies. The glycemic index or GI describes this difference by ranking carbohydrates according to their effect on our blood glucose levels. Choosing low GI carbs—the ones that produce only small fluctuations in our blood glucose and insulin levels—is the secret to good long-term health, thereby reducing your risk of heart disease and diabetes and is the key to sustainable weight loss.

What are the Benefits of the Glycemic Index?

Eating a lot of high GI foods can be detrimental to your health because it pushes your body to extremes. This is especially true if you are overweight and sedentary. Switching to eating mainly low GI carbs, that slowly trickle glucose into your blood stream, keeps your energy levels balanced and means you will feel fuller for longer between meals.

- Low GI diets help people lose and control weight
- Low GI diets increase the body's sensitivity to insulin
- Low GI carbs improve diabetes control
- Low GI carbs reduce the risk of heart disease
- Low GI carbs reduce blood cholesterol levels
- Low GI carbs can help you manage the symptoms of PCOS
- Low GI carbs reduce hunger and keep you fuller for longer

- Low GI carbs prolong physical endurance
- High GI carbs help re-fuel carbohydrates stores after exercise.

How to Switch to a Low GI Diet

The basic technique for eating the low GI way is simply a "this for that" approach—i.e., swapping high GI carbs for low GI carbs. You don't need to count numbers or do any sort of mental arithmetic to make sure you are eating a healthy, low GI diet.

- Use breakfast cereals based on oats, Dalia, Whole wheat bread or Missi Roti or vegetable stuffed roti avoid 'Flakes'.
- Use breads with wholegrains (stone-ground flour)
- Reduce the amount of potatoes you eat
- Enjoy all other types of fruits and vegetables
- Use Basmati or Doongara rice
- Enjoy wheat pasta, Atta noodles
- Eat plenty of salad vegetables

This is the definitive table for both the glycemic index and the glycemic load.

GI of 55 is low; GL of 10 is low.

The Glycemic Index (GI) is a numerical system of measuring how much of a rise in circulating blood sugar a carbohydrate triggers-the higher the number, the greater the blood sugar response. So a low GI food will cause a small rise, while a high GI food will trigger a dramatic spike. A list of carbohydrates with their glycemic values is shown below.

A GI of 70 or more is high.

A GI of 56 to 69 inclusive is medium,

and a GI of 55 or less is low.

The Glycemic Load (GL) is a relatively new way to assess the impact of carbohydrate consumption that takes the glycemic index into account, but gives a fuller picture than

does glycemic index alone. A GI value tells you only how rapidly a particular carbohydrate turns into sugar. It doesn't tell you how much of that carbohydrate is in a serving of a particular food. You need to know both things to understand a food's effect on blood sugar. That is where glycemic load comes in.

The carbohydrate in watermelon, for example, has a high GI. But there isn't a lot of it, so watermelon's glycemic load is relatively low. A GL of 20 or more is high, a GL of 11 to 19 inclusive is medium, and a GL of 10 or less is low.

Foods that have a low GL almost always have a low GI. Foods with an intermediate or high GL range from very low to very high GI.

The GI is of foods based on the glucose index where glucose is set to equal 100. The other is the **glycemic load, which is** the **glycemic index** divided by **100** multiplied by its available **carbohydrate content** (i.e. carbohydrates *minus* fibre) in grams.

Take, watermelon as an example of calculating glycemic load. Its glycemic index is pretty high, about 72. According to the calculations in a serving of 120 grams it has 6 grams of available carbohydrate per serving, so its glycemic load is pretty low, 72/100 6=4.32, rounded to 4.

30 Things You Should Know About Managing Diabetes

Insulin

1. No, the insulin injection doesn't really hurt. Most needles used for insulin injections are small and thin, some as tiny as five-sixteenths of an inch in length, causing little or no pain.
2. It's not unusual for type 2 diabetes persons to need insulin. You may need to add insulin to your regimen to adequately control your blood glucose. It doesn't mean that you've "failed" at managing your condition.
3. There's a right way to do it. Always wash your hands first and wipe the top of the insulin vial with alcohol. Be sure to follow the directions for mixing your insulin if it's NPH. Tap the syringe to remove any air bubbles. It is also critical to mix NPH well in an insulin pen. And if you have a pen, remember that 5-second rule: Keep the thumb button pressed and the needle under the skin for 5 seconds to make sure all the insulin has gone in. Pen or syringe, remember to always inject at a 90-degree angle.
4. Cold insulin has a bite. Using insulin right out of the refrigerator is more likely to hurt than using insulin at room temperature. Insulin in use should be stored at room temperature.
5. Remember that when the muscles near the injection site are exercised shortly before or after a shot, it will increase absorption rate.

Blood Glucose Monitoring

1. All meters are not created equal. Since features of blood glucose meters vary quite a bit, do some research and check with your doctor and diabetes educator before you buy.
2. Accuracy matters. Be sure to use the control solution that comes with your meter, in order to test the meter's accuracy before checking your blood glucose.
3. Meters are often free it's the strips that'll cost you. Often, you will be able to get a free blood glucose meter from your health care team, by rebate from the manufacturer, or from your health insurance company. The test strips are another matter they can be pricey, and you may need to check how many per day your insurance will cover.
4. Monitoring works. Really. Ask your health care team whether and how often you should check your blood glucose. If you have type 2, your recommended monitoring frequency will vary depending upon your overall level of control and the medications you take to treat your diabetes.
5. Even in the digital age, written records help. You may have a meter that stores data electronically, but it's still a good idea to write down your results, along with date and time, and other variables as well, like food, exercise, alcohol, and stress. You can then share this important information with your health care providers or doctor.

Hypoglycemia and Hyperglycemiac

1. Hyper = high, hypo = low. In other words, hyperglycemia means there is too much glucose in the blood, hypoglycemia means there is too little.
2 Lows need glucose, highs need insulin (or exercise). Know the difference, because administering insulin to someone (or yourself) during a low will cause even lower

blood glucose. For type 2s, exercising can help bring down post-meal highs.

3. Symptoms vary. Hypoglycemia is usually characterized by sweating and shaking, a pounding heart, nervousness or irritability, or feeling weak, hungry, tingly, or confused. If you no longer have these warning signs, you are said to have hypoglycemia unawareness, which increases the risk of severe hypoglycemia. If you think you may have hypoglycemia unawareness, talk to your doctor about how to address this. Hyperglycemia, on the other hand, can cause headache, blurry vision, thirst, frequent urination, and dry skin. When in doubt, check your glucose level.
4. If you are experiencing hypoglycemia, take 15 grams of carbohydrate, then check your blood glucose again in 15 minutes. Repeat until you get back up to 70 mg/dl. If you are more than an hour away from a meal, you should probably go ahead and eat at least a small meal to ensure that hypoglycemia does not recur.
5. If your blood glucose is too low, you will need help from others around you. That's why you have to tell family, friends, and co-workers how to recognize a low and help you treat it. Talk to your doctor about whether you need to keep a glucagon kit on hand, and if so, make sure the people around you know how to use it. Call your doctor if you have multiple mild lows or any severe low. And wear an ID that indicates you have diabetes.

Medications

1. When it comes to type 2 medicines, one size does not fit all. There are six different classes of oral agents for type 2: alpha-glucosidase inhibitors, biguanides (metformin), DPP-4 inhibitors, meglitinides, sulfonylureas, and thiazolidinediones or TZDs. Some manufacturers produce combination drugs that combine multiple type 2 drugs into one pill.

2. Older is sometimes better. The newest advances aren't always the best options for everyone. You may be better off with good old metformin than with the newest drug on the market don't be afraid to ask your doctor about your options.
3. You're an individual, not a statistic. Medications have different effects on different people. If you think something about your diabetes, for example, hypoglycemia unawareness may affect what drugs will work for you, then you may be right. Be sure to discuss those things with your health care provider/doctor.
3. It's not a good idea to play doctor. Never discontinue a medication without speaking with your health care provider first. Be sure to talk to your diabetes care provider/doctor about any problems you might be experiencing, and find out what medications are right for you.
4. Your pharmacist is your friend. BUT, insist on proper bill/ receipt with batch numbers.

Your Kidneys

1. Damaged filters don't do the job. HIgh blood glucose over long periods of time damages the kidneys. If this condition progresses, then they don't filter the blood properly, and may eventually fail altogether.
2. Eventually, kidney damage can lead to kidney failure. It's important to remember that for the most part, there are no signs or symptoms of pending kidney failure until kidney disease is already in advanced stages. This is why it's important to keep up with annual screenings.
3. Once a year, your doctor should perform a urine test to check for microalbumin in your urine, which if positive, indicates leakage of protein by the kidneys. This is an early sign of damage to the kidney by diabetes and/or high blood pressure. Your doctor may order other urine

and blood tests to check how well your kidneys are functioning.

4. Kidney failure means dialysis or a transplant. That's why it's so important to keep up with kidney function screenings before kidney failure occurs.
5. There's a lot you can do. Maintain good blood glucose control and good blood pressure levels, avoid high-protein diets, and have your doctor check your kidney function regularly. Blood pressure lowering drugs like ACE inhibitors and ARBs can slow the progress of kidney disease. Blood pressure control is especially important for people with high albumin levels in the urine (microalbuminuria and albuminuria).

Your Eyes

1. In young and middle-aged Indians, most new blindness is due to diabetes. Retinopathy, the most common diabetic eye disease, can lead to blindness.
2. Visit your eye doctor every year for dilated eye and visual exams not just to check your vision, but also to check for diabetic eye diseases like retinopathy.
3. Healthy blood glucose levels are like carrots: Both are good for your eyes. Keeping up with blood glucose management lowers the risk of developing eye disease and keeps existing eye disease from getting worse.
4. It's worse under pressure. High blood pressure can cause damage to blood vessels in the eye, and can made diabetic eye disease worse. Talk to your doctor about ways to control your blood pressure.
5. Cholesterol counts. High cholesterol can also cause damage to blood vessels in the eye. Keep cholesterol down to keep eye disease from developing or worsening.

Indian Ethnicity Tied to Higher Diabetes Risk

New York (Reuters Health)—Americans of Indian descent may have a heightened risk of diabetes, even when their weight is in the normal range, research suggests.

Researchers found that among more than 7,400 Asian Americans in a national health study, *those of Indian descent had roughly three times the risk of diabetes as U.S. whites as a whole, and a higher prevalence of the disease than people of other Asian ethnicities.*

Moreover, although type 2 diabetes is closely associated with obesity, Asian Indians' risk began to climb even at lower weights.

Among those with weights in the normal range—as measured by Body Mass Index (BMI), a ratio of weight in relation to height—about 7 per cent had diabetes. That compared with rates of anywhere from 2 per cent to 4 per cent among whites and people of other Asian ethnicities.

Among obese adults—as defined as a BMI of 30 or higher—one-third of Indian adults had diabetes. Among other ethnicities, the rate ranged from 12 per cent to 17 per cent.

The reasons for the findings are not entirely clear. However, the researchers note, ethnic differences in body fat levels and body fat distribution may play a role.

Studies have shown that compared with people of other races and ethnicities, Asians tend to have a higher proportion of body fat at any given weight—along with a higher type 2 diabetes risk.

It's possible that people of Indian background are particularly likely to have body fat distributions—including more abdominal fat—that are closely associated with diabetes, according to Oza-Frank and colleagues.

Some studies, the researchers note, have suggested that this may be a factor in the higher diabetes risk seen in Indian adults compared with Europeans.

Because Asian adults tend to have more body fat—and, therefore, greater health risks at relatively lower weights—the World Health Organization (WHO) has proposed lowering the threshold for how "overweight" is defined in Asian populations.

The standard definition of overweight is a BMI of between 25 and 30; the WHO recommendation sets that at 23 to 27.5 for Asians.

This needs for more research into the "complex relationships" among body size, body fat and disease risks across different Asian populations.

Which Nut is the Best and Healthiest?

A new study positions walnuts in the No. 1 slot among a family of foods that lay claim to being among the most nearly perfect, packaged foods and it only takes 7 walnuts a day to get the benefits....

In a report at the 241st National Meeting and Exposition of the American Chemical Society, scientists presented an analysis showing that walnuts have a combination of more healthful antioxidants and higher quality antioxidants than any other nut.

Joe Vinson, Ph.D., who did the analysis stated that, "Walnuts rank above peanuts, almonds, pecans, pistachios and other nuts." "A handful of walnuts contains almost twice as much antioxidants as an equivalent amount of any other commonly consumed nut. But unfortunately, people don't eat a lot of them. This study suggests that consumers should eat more walnuts as part of a healthy diet."

Vinson noted that nuts in general have an unusual combination of nutritional benefits—in addition to those antioxidants—wrapped into a convenient and inexpensive package. Nuts, for instance, contain plenty of high-quality protein that can substitute for meat; vitamins and minerals; dietary fibre; and are dairy—and gluten-free. Years of research by scientists around the world link regular consumption of small amounts of nuts or peanut butter with decreased risk of heart disease, certain kinds of cancer, gallstones, Type 2 diabetes, and other health problems.

Despite all the previous research, scientists until now had not compared both the amount and quality of antioxidants found in different nuts, Vinson said. He filled that knowledge gap by analyzing antioxidants in nine different types of nuts: walnuts, almonds, peanuts, pistachios, hazelnuts, Brazil nuts, cashews, and pecans. Walnuts had the highest levels of antioxidants.

Vinson also found that the quality, or potency of antioxidants present in walnuts was highest among the nuts. Antioxidants in walnuts were 2-15 times as potent as vitamin E, renowned for its powerful antioxidant effects that protect the body against damaging natural chemicals involved in causing disease.

"There's another advantage in choosing walnuts as a source of antioxidants," said Vinson, who is with the University of Scranton in Pennsylvania. "The heat from roasting nuts generally reduces the quality of the antioxidants. People usually eat walnuts raw or unroasted, and get the full effectiveness of those antioxidants."

If nuts are so healthful and nutritious, why don't people eat more?

Vinson's research shows, for instance, that nuts account for barely 8 per cent of the daily antioxidants in the average person's diet. Many people may not be aware that nuts are such a healthful food. Others may be concerned about gaining weight from a food so high in fat and calories. But he points out that nuts contain healthful polyunsaturated and monosaturated fats rather than artery-clogging saturated fat. As for the calories, eating nuts does not appear to cause weight gain and even makes people feel full and less likely to overeat. In a 2009 U.S. study, nut consumption was associated with a significantly lower risk of weight gain and obesity. Still, consumers should keep the portion size small. Vinson said it takes only about 7 walnuts a day, for instance, to get the potential health benefits uncovered in previous studies.

Dining Out with Diabetes

The more active the role you play in your health-care decisions, the easier it is to manage your diabetes. For instance, cooking your own meals allows for better blood-sugar control because you known extactly what and how much is in your food. However, it's not always possible to prepare home-cooked meals. And living with diabetes doesn't mean you can't enjoy dining out.

Follow These Tips for Smart Dining : Plan Ahead

- Choose a restaurant with a large menu of healthy items. Many chains have nutritional information available online.
- Call the restaurant ahead of time and ask whether they can handle special requests.
- Have a small snack before going to a restaurant, when you are dining later than usual, so you aren't too hungry.
- Review your meal plan before going out, so you will know what your carbohydrate allocation is.

Ordering Meals

- If you aren't sure how a dish is prepared, ask your server.
- Watch your portion sizes. For the main course, order an appetizer and either split an entrée with your companion or eat half of it and take the rest home.
- Ask for substitutions. For example, order vegetables instead of French fries.
- Avoid breaded, fried foods and foods in heavy sauces. Try fish or poultry that's grilled or broiled, without butter.

- Ask for salad dressing and sauces on the side.
- Limit to one serving drink that contain alcohol.
- Be careful of all-you-can-eat restaurants. When you do eat at a buffet, fill up first on vegetable dishes.

With these tips in mind, you can keep your blood glucose in control and make dining out an enjoyable experience.

Foods to be Avoided

Low Protein — Low Sugar

Foods to be avoided

1. Extra Milk or Milk Products, Fish, Chicken and Egg.
2. Pulses and Legumes.
3. Fried Foods, e.g. Puri, Pakora, Parantha, Samosa.
4. Sugar, Sweets, Gur, Honey, Glucose, Jam, Jelly, Sweet, Chutney etc.
5. Dry Fruits, e.g. Peanuts, Kishmish, Cashewnuts, Coconut, Khajur etc.
6. Fruit Juices, Colas, Aerated Drinks, Sherbets, Complan, Squashes.
7. Alcohol and Beer.
8. Egg Yolk, Seafood, Cream, Cheese (Paneer), Ghee, Organ Meat.
9. Fruits—Mango, Litchi, Grapes, Cheeku, Banana, Sharifa, Musk-Melon Lemon, Orange, Mausmi, Apricots.
10. Salted Butter.
11. Salted Dry fruits and Namkeens
12. Papad, Chutney, Pickles.
13. No Baking Soda to be used in Cooking.
14. No Salt permitted at the table.
15. Avoid Breads or Other Baked products.
16. All the Canned Products.
17. Pulses like Bengal Gram Dal, Lentil.
18. Antacids—ENO etc.
19. Coconut Water, Jaljeera, Pudina Pani.

NO FAST NO FEAST

Low Sodium — Low Sugar

Foods to be avoided

1. Fried foods, e.g. Puri, Pakora, Parantha, Samosa.
2. Sugar, Sweets, Gur, Honey, Glucose, Jam, Jelly, Sweet, Chutney etc.
3. Dry Fruits, e.g. Peanuts, Kishmish, Cashewnuts, Coconut, Khajur etc.
4. Fruit Juices, Colas, Aerated Drinks, Sherbets, Bournvita.
5. Alcohol and Beer.
6. Whole Milk, Cream, Cheese (Paneer), Ghee, Organ Meat, Egg yolk, Seafood.
7. Fruits—Mango, Litchi, Grapes, Cheeku, Banana, Sharifa, Musk Melon, Lemon.
8. Vegetables—Aloo, Arbi, Jimikand, Shakarkandi, Beetroot, Green Leafy Vegetables—Methi, Bathua, Lettuce, Dhania, Ganth Gobhi, Lotus Stems, Radish, Carrot, Spinach (Once a Week).
9. Salt Preserved Fish or Meats.
10. Salted Butter.
11. Salted Dry Fruits or Namkeens (esp.).
12. Papad, Chutney, Pickles.
13. Avoid Breads or Other Baked Products.
14. All the Canned Products.
15. Pulses like Bengal Gram Dal, Lentil.
16. Antacids—ENO etc.
17. Coconut Water, Jaljeera, Pudina Pani.
18. No Baking Soda to be used in Cooking.
19. No Salt permitted at the Table.

Others

1. Never Have Alcohol on Empty Stomach.
2. Mix Chana or Bajra or Jowar Flour to Wheat Flour (1 : 3).
3. Methi Dana Soaked Seeds Along with Water can be taken.
4. Avoid Fasting or Skipping or Meals.
5. Follow a Regular Exercise Plan.

Exchanges for one chapati

1 Chapati = ½ Katori Cooked Rice / Upma / Dalia / Kichri / Poha / Oats or 30 gms Bhuna Chana / Murmura / Popcorn / Sevian / Sabutdana / Cornflakes or 4-5 Marrie Biscuits / 2 Monaco Biscuits / 1 Rusk / 1 Brown Bread Slice / 1 Idli / 1 Plain Dosa.

Free Vegetables

Karela, Brinjal, Onion, Pumpkin, Cucumber, Tinda, French Beans, Ladies Finger, Drumstick, Turnip, Mushrooms, Tomato.

Household Measures

1 Table Spoon = 15 gms, 1 Tea spoon = 5 gms, 1 Katori = 200 ml, 1 Glass = 250 ml, 1 Cup = 150 ml

"Avoid" Foods

Try and avoid use of direct sugar in foods.
Many people use recipes or buy ready to eat foods. Any such recipe or food label, which calls for the use of following food items usually means that direct sugars have been added and should be avoided.

Foods to avoid

brown sugar
corn sweetener
corn syrup
fructose
fruit juice concentrate
glucose (dextrose)
high-fructose corn syrup
honey
invert sugar
lactose
maltose
molasses
raw sugar
[table] sugar (sucrose) syrup

Free Foods

These are foods which have less than 5 gms. of carbohydrates

They can be used to appease hunger in case you are on a diet which makes you feel very hungry even after you have eaten the serving allowed in the meal.

At the same time, not more than 2-3 servings of food which have their portion size listed should be eaten in day otherwise the carbohydrates and calories in these food items would need to be considered as a part of the food servings allowed in your diet plan.

Foods Serving Sizes Made Easy

The servings (sizes and quantities) of each food item in anyone group is determined such that they provide the standard amount of these three nutrients (and consequently, calories) which have been defined for each food group.

Weight:	1 ounce = 30 gms (in reality 28.25 gms)
Volume:	1 level tea spoon = 5 ml; 1 level table spoon =15 ml 1 fluid ounce = 30 ml; 1 cup = 140 ml = 8 fluid ounces.
Length:	1 inch = 2.5 cms (in reality 2.54 cms)

Many people feel uncomfortable with weighing and measuring foods. Frankly, within a few days you will get a very good visual grasp of the amounts and will not really have to bother about the precise weights and volumes.

Moreover, here are some household measures which will give you a better idea about quantity and how you will estimate the weights and volumes.

Food portions (tips and tricks)

1 teaspoon (5ml)

About the size of the top half of your thumb

25 gm of flour (atta) is approximate what can be held in an average Indian woman palm

1 ounce (28 g)

approximately a inch cube of cheese

volume of four stacked dice

slice of cheese is about the size of a 3-1/2 inch computer disk

chunk of cheese is about as thick as 2 dominoes

1 handful (palm) of nuts

2 ounces (57 g)

1 small chicken leg or thigh

1/2 cup of cottage cheese or tuna

3 ounces (85 g)

serving of meat is about the size of a deck of playing cards (3 exchanges)

1/2 of whole chicken breast

1 medium pork chop

1 small hamburger

undreaded fish fillet

1/2 cup (118 ml)

fruit or vegetables can fit in the palm or your hand
about the volume of a tennis ball

1 cup (236 ml)

about the size of a woman's fist

breakfast cereal goes halfway up the side of a standard cereal bowl

broccoli is about the size of a light bulb

1 medium apple = A tennis ball

Foods to be Avoided

Foods to be avoided	Foods to be included
- **Whole milk**	- Toned milk and curd
- Fried foods- Puri, Pakora, Parantha, Namkeens etc.	- Roasted namkeens or baked snacks
- Egg yolk, Red meats, Organ meats- eg. liver, kidney etc.	White of egg/fish, Chicken/ paneer (only 2) (60-70 gms) (30gms)
- Sugar, Gur, Honey, Glucose	- Equal or sugar free
- Sweet items-chocolates, jam, jelly, ice-creams, mithai, cakes, pastries etc.	- Sugar free products
- Dry fruits—peanuts, kishmish, coconut, cashewnuts, khajur etc.	
- Butter, Ghee, Cream, Cheese	- Refined oil-limited amounts
- Drinks like-Fruit juices, cold drinks, sherbets, complan, cream soups	- Veg. Juice, Lemon water, soda, coke Lassi, Clear soups, Jaljeera, Gingerale, Ambi-pana
- Few vegetables— Aloo, arbi, jimikand, shakarkandi, beetroot	- Free vegetables-Salads and green leafy vegetables
- Few fruits— Mango, lichi, grapes, cheeku, banana, sharifa	- All the others (100-200 gms)
- All alcoholic drinks	

Role of Fibre in Diabetes

Dietary fibre and complex carbohydrate benefit types I and II diabetes. Such diets lower

1. Insulin requirements.
2. Increase peripheral tissue insulin sensitivity.
3. Decrease serum cholesterol and triglyceride level.
4. Aid in weight control.
5. Lowers blood pressure.

Soluble fibres such as pectin, gums, hemicelluloses (in fruits), increase intestinal transit time, Delay gastric emptying, slow glucose absorption and lowers serum cholesterol.

Insoluble fibres such as cellulose and lignin (vegetables, grains) decrease intestinal transit time, increase faecal bulk, and delay glucose absorption and slow starch hydrolysis.

Diets high in fibres and carbohydrates improve glucose metabolism without increasing insulin secretion. High fibre diet promotes weight loss. They increase satiety, delay gastric emptying by releasing certain gut hormones. With high fibre foods starch, fatty acids may be less well absorbed.

Fenugreek seeds, which contain high fibre, are useful to diabetics. It contains mucilaginous fibre and total fibre to an extent of 20 per cent and 50 per cent repectively. In addition it also contains trigonelline—an alkaloid known to reduce blood sugar level.

Recommended daily intake of fibre is 30-40 grams.

Fibre content of Indian foods (per 100 grams)

Contents	Grams
Barley	3.9
Ragi	3.6
Wheat flour (whole)	1.9
Wheat flour (refined)	0.3
Wheat bread (white)	0.2
Bengal gram (whole)	3.9
Bengal gram (dal)	1.2
Green gram	4.1
Soybean	3.7
Red gram	6.2
Amaranth	1.0
Betel leaves	2.3
Cabbage	1.0
Colocasia leaves	2.9
Curry leaves	1.2
Drumstick leaves	6.4
Fenugreek leaves	1.1
Potato	0.4
Onion	0.6
Radish	o.6
Karela	1.7
Brinjal	1.3
Broad beans	2.0
Cluster beans	3.2
Drumstick	4.8
Parwar	3.0
Coconut dry	6.6
Coconut fresh	3.6
Gingelly seeds	2.9
Groundnut	3.1
Amla	3.4

Contents	Grams
Apple	1.0
Banana	0.4
Grapes	2.8
Guava	5.2
Mango	0.7
Orange	0.3
Papaya	0.8
Pineapple	0.5

Alcohol and Diabetes

1. Alcohol contributes to empty calories and upset the dietary regulation.
2. Alcohol damages the liver. Hypoglycemia occurs due to impairment of glucose generating capacity of liver. Alcohol is absorbed from the stomach and reaches the liver through blood stream. It is metabolized and the capacity to release glucose from its reserve stores is blocked. Thus, the danger of lowering of blood sugar levels is there in diabetics.
3. Alcohol induced intoxication may mask the usual symptoms of low blood glucose levels.
4. Combination of alcohol and sulphonylurea may cause intense palpitation and flushing of face.
5. Alcohol should be avoided if obesity, hypertension, hypertriglyceridemia is present.

Energy value of hard and soft drinks

Drink	*Amount*	*Calories*
Beer	140ml	127
Brandy	30ml	77
Gin	43ml	105
Rum	43ml	105
Whisky	43ml	105
Wine	43ml	105
Pepsi	1 Bottle	84
Fanta	1 Bottle	84
Limca	1 Bottle	52
Thumsup	1 Bottle	84
Coke	1 Bottle	84

- **Health Hazards: Excessive alcohol intake** contributes to obesity, high blood pressure, stroke, heart and liver disease, some cancers, and even impotence. **Concentration and short-term memory** are reduced as well as athletic performance.
  Other alcohol hazards include: Fetal Alcohol Syndrome, stomach upsets, menstrual problems, depression, snoring sleep problems, work absenteeism, impaired judgement, and social/family problems.
- **Alcohol contributes to obesity:** Through its high calories and by lessening the body's ability to burn fat. Fat storage is promoted, particularly in the belly—a health danger zone. Alcohol can also stimulate the appetite.
- **Alcohol is potentially more harmful while dieting:** Blood sugar levels may drop with resultant fatigue and further impairment of concentration, reflexes and driving skills—and maybe even the dieter's resolve!

Lower Risk Alcohol Limits

Women: No more than 1 drink per day.
Men: No more than 2 drinks per day (Over 65 ml drink)
(At least 2 days a week should be alcohol-free)

	12 fl.oz Regular Beer (5% Alc.)
1 Drink Contains	OR 14 fl.oz Light Beer (4.2% Alc.)
14 grams Alcohol:	OR 5 fl.oz Wine (12% Alc.)
	OR 1½ fl.oz Spirits (80 Proof)

Note : You cannot save daily drinks for one occasion. Binge drinking is particularly harmful: 4 drinks for males or 3 drinks for females (within 2 hours).

For some people, safe drinking means no alcohol at all. Even one drink may impair driving skills, particularly if tired. For women who drink frequently, breast cancer risk is increased by 9 per cent for each drink after the first drink.

It is advisable not to drink at all if you are:

- pregnant, trying to conceive or breastfeeding

- taking medication or have liver or heart disease (unless approved by your doctor or pharmacist)
- planning to drive, use machinery or play sports
- studying or needing to concentrate
- a child or adolescent.

- Women and adolescents are more prone to alcohol's ill-effects due to their lower body weight, smaller livers and lesser capacity to metabolize alcohol. As we age, our ability to handle alcohol decreases.
- Excess alcohol contributes to obesity, high blood pressure and many other health problems

How to Calculate Alcohol Content

Per cent alcohol on label refers to alcohol volume (ml alcohol/ 100 ml). Note: 100ml = 3½ fl.oz

To convert to grams (weight) of alcohol, multiply the per cent volume by 0.8—since 1 ml of alcohol weighs only 0.8 grams.

Example—12 fl.oz Can Beer (5% alcohol)
5% alc. volume = 5% of 12 fl.oz = 0.6 fl.oz
= 18ml alcohol (Note: 1 fl.oz = 30 ml)
Weight (18ml × 0.8) = 14.4g alcohol.

Alcohol
Should We or Should We Not...

Just a Drop of Common Sense

After you are diagnosed with diabetes, you might find yourself learning quite a bit about your diet. Much of this involves making decisions about how best to eat and drink to achieve good outcomes and avoid problems with your therapy. While some rules are fairly obvious, for others, far less evidence is available. One such example is drinking alcohol.

Let's face it: Alcohol is a potent drug that can have a profound, and often negative, impact on users. Still, millions of people in India drink alcohol on a regular basis, and many of them have diabetes. The prevailing wisdom was that alcohol could impair your judgment, make it difficult to sense the onset of hypoglycemia, and inhibit self-management. While there wasn't much experimental evidence supporting these assertions, it was the party line of the time.

Today, however, increasing evidence suggests that moderate consumption has many beneficial effects for people with diabetes. In a comprehensive review of several studies on the effect of alcohol use by people with diabetes, the data show that *drinking heavily (i.e., more than three drinks per day) can have more deleterious effects on health status than does moderate consumption.* Indeed, moderate alcohol intake (i.e., one to two drinks per day) is associated with decreased incidence of coronary heart disease, a major killer of people with type 2 diabetes; improved lipids; and, potentially, reduction of inflammatory response, which is increasingly linked to the risk of cardiovascular disease events.

Limited research also suggests that alcohol is not associated with adverse outcomes when using diabetes tablets. Moderate consumption was found to have no acute effects on blood sugar control in type 2 diabetes. In type 1, it may in fact cause hypoglycemia the following morning, and the usual symptons of hypoglycemia may be masked and impair the counter-regulatory responses for normalisation.

This suggests that people with type 1 need to consider diet regulation when they drink and make sure they are monitoring their blood glucose.

While moderate consumption of alcohol may have some positive benefits for those who already drink, the science does not support adding alcohol to your diet if you don't currently do so.

But if you have diabetes and you do drink, it is important to discuss this with your health team. Make them aware that drinking alcohol is part of your lifestyle and that you want to continue to do so in a responsible fashion. A dietitian can show you how to enjoy a glass of wine or beer with your meals without adding excessive calories.

Optimal control of diabetes is not only about attaining good Lab report numbers, but achieving a lifestyle that is comfortable and rewarding while you do so. You can, with a little thought, drink a glass of fine wine with your meal and by doing so benefit your health—and your enjoyment of life.

Frequently Asked Questions

Questions—Answers

Q.1. Do artificial sweeteners have any harmful effect?

Ans. There are no medical grounds to indicate that when consumed in moderation Artificial sweeteners cause any health hazard. Available artificial sweeteners are of two types :

(a) Nutritive sweeteners, having same calories as sugar, e.g. Sorbitol, fructose.

(b) Non-nutritive sweeteners, e.g. Saccharin, aspartame. The latter are being used now-a-days.

Q.2. What kinds of fruit can diabetic take?

Ans. Diabetics can take those fruits, which do not have high free sugar content. Sweet fruits like mango, banana, and grapes should be restricted. Instead citrus fruits like papaya, guava, apple are permitted.

Q.3. Can diabetics take desserts?

Ans. Yes, provided calories from desserts are worked out into daily schedule and use of free sugar in their preparation is avoided.

Q.4. Can diabetics take rice?

Ans. Yes, but as rice contains refined carbohydrate up to 75 per cent its absorption is fast so there is quick rise of blood glucose. Therefore, rice should be preferably taken mixed with soybean, bengal gram, rajma etc.

Q.5. Is milk good for diabetics?

Ans. Skimmed or low fat milk is recommended to diabetics. Cream, condensed milk, khoya need to be avoided. Curd, yoghurt, buttermilk can be included in the diet.

Q.6. Can diabetics take alcohol?

Ans. It is better for diabetics to avoid alcohol. Alcohol has empty calories that cannot be metabolized in the system. After few drinks, a person tends to eat more liberally, so caloric restriction is not possible. Alcohol consumption over a period of time can damage liver in diabetic and lead to cirrhosis. So diabetic is advised to refrain from alcohol.

Q.7. Which cooking oil is recommended for diabetes?

Ans. Diabetics are more prone to heart diseases and it is essential that they keep their Blood cholesterol and triglycerides level at a normal level. Total calories from fat in the diet of a diabetic should be less than 20-30 per cent. The following cooking oil with low content of saturated fats is recommended: safflower, sunflower, soybean oil, and corn oil, til oil, groundnut oil, or mustard oil.

Q.8. Does the method of preparation of food make difference in total caloric value of meal ?

Ans. Method of preparation plays an important role in total calories value of food, some examples of low calorie preparation, are (a) meat stew compared to meat curry; (b) boiled or poached egg compared to fried egg or omelette; (c) baked vegetables to fried or curried vegetable.

Q.9. What is advised regarding salad dressings, to be used for diabetics?

Ans. Dressings should be of fresh lime, vinegar or curd. Mayonaise, salad oil, French dressings are to be avoided.

Q.10. Have spices any nutritive value?

Ans. Spices have some minerals and trace elements. These are added to food in very small amounts as to bring out flavour and taste in meal prepared.

Q.11. Which is a better diet, vegetarian or non-vegetarian?

Ans. Vegetarian diets are preferred as animal sources are rich in saturated fats which should be avoided.

Q.12. What is the right time for injecting an insulin injection?

Ans. Insulin injection should be taken 1/2 hour before meal and there should be a difference of 12 hours in between two injections. Huminsulin reacts immediately so it can be taken just before the meal.

Q.13. Can insulin dosage be adjusted with the amount of food taken for example, when going to party or taking less food?

Ans. Yes, if you feel that you will have less or no food today then you can decrease your insulin dosage and *vice versa* if you think that you cannot control your intake in a party.

Q.14. Does insulin injection causes weight gain ?

Ans. Uncontrolled diabetes causes weight loss, but as soon as it is controlled your weight tends to be stable or there is weight gain. If a person is on insulin, he feels more hungry and hence weight gain is seen in some.

Q.15. How often can we have cold drinks or tea?

Ans. Tea can be taken twice or thrice without sugar in a day. Cold drinks should be avoided as they contain calories. Pepsi or coke can be taken occasionally.

Q.16. What precautions should be taken while eating out?

Ans. While eating out, refrain from eating very oily and rich food. If there is choice, reach out for boiled, grilled or baked food instead. Avoid rich gravies. Clear soups should be preferred. Plain lime juice or soda is better than cold drinks or shakes.

Boiled rice, plain roti should be preferred to biryanis, pulaos, puri, parantha etc. Salads without dressing should be taken. Fruits can be taken as desserts.

Q.17. Can diabetics take dry fruits ?

Ans. Dry fruits like raisins, coconut, etc. are not permitted to diabetics.

Q.18. How many nuts can be included in a diabetic diet?

Ans. These are allowed as exchange food, the equivalent of 100 kcal being substitute for one cup skimmed milk, one slice bread or chapati for normal weight diabetic and for obese diabetics this exchange should be substituted by his/her fat exchange.

Three walnuts, 10-12 almonds, 16-20 groundnuts, 15-20 pistachios, or 8 cashewnuts provide 100 kcal.

Exercise

Exercise!!!

When your doctor tells you to exercise, he is saying nothing new. More than 2000 years back, Charak, in his Charak Samhita, advocated the use of exercise in treating diabetes. In fact, the use of exercise in the treatment of diabetes was prescribed as early as 600 BC by the Indian physician Sushruta, and was widely recommended by physicians of the 18th century. Elliot Joslin, often called the Father of modern diabetes, identified exercise along with dietary management and insulin administration as one of the three components of good therapy in the 1920s.

It could be argued that in the absence of any other forms of treatment, the older day physicians had no choice but to fall back on diet and exercise! Later, with the wide availability of oral hypoglycemic agents and insulin, the relative importance of exercise as a treatment for diabetes seemed to go into a decline from which it is just emerging.

With the long-term safety and efficacy of some of the oral agents being called into question and with reports that ill advised insulin therapy leading to high blood insulin levels can be a factor in leading to many disorders such as high blood pressure, lipid disorders and even atherosclerosis, attention is being again given to diet and exercise as the dominant treatment modalities, as far as possible.

If a diabetic can be managed with the use of diet and exercise alone, or if the addition of exercise can lead to a substantial decrease in the dose of the oral agent or the insulin, can thereby any justification for not prescribing exercise to the diabetics!

It is well documented that for every mile that you jog, you add one minute to your life.

Exercise.......Why?

But who like to exercise, and too regularly. In the modern age where even the routine activity in daily life has been decreased due to the availability of modern gadgets and conveniences, exercise for many is the use of one's thumb to press the "Remote Control" button!

But...the benefits from a regular exercise schedule are tremendous for all people, but for people with diabetes specifically include:

- It helps in lowering the blood glucose levels. The reason for this is that muscles which are working use more glucose than those that are resting. Muscle movement leads to greater sugar uptake by muscle cells and lower blood sugar levels. Moreover, the sensitivity to insulin is increased, so that more glucose is allowed to enter the cells and be utilised, again leading to a decrese in blood glucose levels.
- Improved insulin sensitivity. The increase in insulin sensitivity is not only related to the loss of weight which occurs in a person who is overweight, but there is evidence to show that insulin sensitivity can increase as much as 40 per cent in a person with diabetes who exercises regularly without a loss of weight!
- As a consequence, there are lower basal and postprandial insulin concentration (especially in type 2 diabetes).
- Lower glycosolated haemoglobin levels, due to the lowering of the blood glucose levels.
- Improved lipid profile. There is a lowering of the serum triglyceride levels. Moreover, there is a reduction of Low Density Lipoprotein cholesterol (LDL), or bad cholesterol, which forms plaque that obstructs blood vessels. Exercise promotes the good cholesterol, High Density Lipoprotein cholesterol (HDL), which is protective against heart disease.

- Blood pressure is also lowered through exercise and exercise has been shown to improve mild to moderate high blood pressure.
- Increased energy expenditure, which allows a person to achieve his optimal body weight. Moreover, exercise reduces the fat in the body and increases the muscle mass.
- Improved fuctioning of the cardiovascular system. Consider the benefits of a well-conditioned heart: In 1 minute with 45 to 50 beats, the heart of a well-conditioned person pumps the same amount of blood as an inactive person's heart pumps in 70 to 75 beats. Compared to the well-conditioned heart, the average heart pumps up to 36,000 more times per day, 13 million more times per year.
- Increased strength and flexibility improved quality of life and self-esteem, and reduced psychological stress.

Do you still need more reasons to exercise ! ! !

Here is a General Checklist which can help you judge your fitness to exercise.

Modified Physical Activity Readiness Questionnaire (PAR-Q) Regular exercise associated with many health benefits, yet any change of activity may increase the risk of injury. Completion of this questionnaire is a first step when planning to increase the amount of physical activity in your life. Please read each question carefully and answer every question honestly:

Yes No (1) Has a physician ever said you have a heart condition and you should only do physical activity recommended by a physician?

Yes No (2) When you do physical activity, do you feel pain in your chest?

Yes No (3) When you were not doing physical activity, have you had chest pain in the past month?

Yes No (4) Do you ever loose consciousness or do you loose your balance because of dizziness?

Yes	No	(5) Do you have a joint or bone problem that may be made worse by a change in your physical activity?
Yes	No	(6) Is a physician currently prescribing medications for your blood pressure or heart condition.
Yes	No	(7) Are you pregnant?
Yes	No	(8) Do you have insulin dependent diabetes?
Yes	No	(9) Are you 55 years of age or older?
Yes	No	(10) Do you know of any other reason you should not exercise or increase your physical activity?

If you answered yes to any of the above questions, talk to your doctor before you become mere physically active. Tell your doctor your intent to exercise and to which questions you answer yes.

If your health changes so you then answer yes to any of the above questions, seek guidance from a physician.

This Checklist is only for general guidance and it would be better for you to discuss your schedule with your doctor before starting on the exercise programme.

Exercise.......The prescription!

But how does one go about exercising? Patients are often told that they must exercise! And many of us accept this. Today, if you went to a doctor with an infection, and were told "Take antibiotics!", would you accept this? Frankly, no doctor would give such advice. The doctor would need to prescribe the precise antibiotic that you would need to take. You would also be told the strength of the tablets, the number of times you have to take the tablets daily, the number of days that the tablets need to be taken, the time of taking the tablets, the relationship with meal times and even the side effects that the patient may experience!

In the same way, it is also essential that you be advised about any special aspects, precautions and side effects associated with this exercise regime.

Exercise......Evaluation

Before undertaking an exercise schedule, you will need to be evaluated for your fitness to exercise.

In my opinion, a good history and clinical examination along with a few routine investigations would tell the doctor if you are at special risk to undertake an exercise programme.

If you have a significant degree of ischemic heart disease, it may be better for you to follow a special cardiac programme for exercise. In case you have been told that you have eye complications such as proliferative retinopathy, then you should avoid vigorous exercise at least until you have been adequately managed by laser therapy. Similarly those with a significant degree of kidney involvement would also do well to avoid any sudden and vigorous activity. The feet of the patients, especially those with a severe degree of anaesthesia and peripheral vascular disease would require special attention. But the vast majority of people with diabetes can well follow an exercise schedule and should be made to do so!

It is needless to say that all diabetics who are put on an exercise programme should be closely monitored at least in the initial stages.

Should all patients have a cardiac stress test before they undertake an exercise schedule?

An exercise stress test may also be helpful to assess the cardiovascular system if an exercise programme of moderate-to-high intensity is to be undertaken and there is high risk for underlying heart disease. It may be better to have a graded stress test if one of the following criteria is present: • age > 35 years • type 2 diabetes of > 10 yesrs' duration • type 1 diabetes of > 15 years' duration • presence of any additional risk factor for coronary artery disease (high cholesterol, high blood pressure, obesity, stress) • presence of microvascular disease (retinopathy, nephropathy, microalbuminuria) • peripheral vascular disease • autonomic neuropathy.

Guidelines for Adjusting Food during Exercising

If your exercise is unplanned, if your blood glucose level is less than 100 - 120 mg/dl or if about 90 minutes have passed since your last meal, increase your food intake. Pre-exercise snacks are recommended.

For mild to moderate exercise of less than 30 minutes...	Eat a snack of approximately 15 grams carbohydrate, such as an 8 oz. glass of low fat milk, half of a banana or a small apple.
For moderate intensity exercise, longer than 60 minutes...	Eat a snack containing roughly 20-30 grams carbohydrate approximately every 45 minutes. *Note*: If you are exercising longer than 60 minutes, it is advised that you check your blood glucose level every 45-60 minutes. This will allow you to make food or medication adjustments as needed. If your blood glucose is 180 or more, you may not need an extra snack for that hour of exercise.
If your exercise is of moderate intensity and longer than 60 minutes...	Sip on a carbohydrate replacement drink.
To offset post-exercise late onset hypoglycemia...	Remember to eat foods that contain slow-releasing, complex carbohydrates to offset post exercise, late-onset hypoglycemia.
If you are exercising to lose weight...	Limit the amount of extra food you need to keep your blood glucose from dropping too low. If you take insulin or oral diabetic medication, check with

	your health care team for guidance on how best to adjust your medication instead of increasing your food.
Always be prepared for low blood glucose....	By carrying a concentrated form of carbohydrate, such as granulated sugar, glucose tablets etc.

LOSE WEIGHT

GAIN LIFE

EAT RIGHT

AND EXERCISE

Exercise and Precautions

Do I need to adjust my medications when I exercise?

Change may be necessary for some of the patients although this may not be something that you would need to do every time you exercise. The reason for this is that, if you have a regular exercise schedule, your diet and medications will have taken this into consideration and will rarely require adjustments. At the same time, you should be aware about the modification that they may have to make during exercise schedule.

It is possible that you may have to carry out a vigorous activity unexpectedly, or on occasion, you may feel like exercising for a more prolonged period, or at a time which is not your usual time for exercise and therefore, this may not have been taken into account while planning the diet and treatment.

It is better to understand the changes which take place when you exercise so that you better comprehend the adjustments which may have to be made by you, if necessary.

When a normal person exercises, the insulin level in his body decreases. At the time, the level of the insulin antagonist hormones, like catecholamines, increases. The levels of glucagon may remain the same, but in view of the fact that there is a decrease in the insulin level, one could consider this as being a relative increase in the glucagon action during exercise. The reason for this is that when a person exercises, the muscles utilise the glucose and there is a need to replenish the blood glucose such that hypoglycemia is averted. This is done through the liver making new glucose and pouring it into the circulation. Insulin inhibits this, whilst glucagon and other antagonist hormones increase the amount of glucose formed by the liver. It is apparent that there is indeed a fine tuning of the balance between insulin and its antagonist hormones so that the blood glucose levels would be maintained within acceptable limits. Although the changes during excercise are definitely much more complicated than this. I have kept the discussion to these simple terms so that the modifications required in the treatment can be self- apparent.

Let us first consider the patient who has just taken his insulin injection. Obviously, his blood insulin levels would be high and since this a insulin which has been injected, there is no way that the body mechanism can decrease the levels of the insulin when exercise commences. These relatively high insulin levels would exert their effect and prevent the liver from forming new glucose. This would be in spite of the increase in the amount of the use up the glucose, the body would not be able to increase blood glucose levels and there would be tendency for the patient to go into hypoglycemia. Whilst this decrease in the levels of the blood glucose is one of the benefits of exercise, in a finely controlled patient, undue exercise could make him severely hypoglycemic.

Thus, it becomes quite apparent that the problem for patients taking insulin would be:

(a) To try and decrease the blood levels of insulin such that this would not inhibit the ability of the liver to form new glucose and thus maintain the blood glucose levels to within acceptable limits.
(b) Increase the intake of carbohydrates so that this would make up the decrease in the capacity of the liver to form new glucose.

How can these problems be managed? This can be quite easily managed by:

(a) decreasing the dose of insulin that the patient takes prior to the exercise;
(b) take additional carbohydrates before, during or after the exercise;
(c) you may have to do all three, if the exercise is sufficiently vigorous and of a long enough duration.

Another way to keep your blood glucose under control while you are exercising to adjust your medication. But before major adjustments to your medication, check with your doctor to ensure you are making the correct decision.

If you take oral drugs	Your physician may suggest that use less medication to keep your blood glucose from going too low during exercise. If your blood glucose falls below 80 mmg/dl after exercise, you will need to decrease your medication. Be sure to test your blood glucose levels to know for sure where you stand.
If you use insulin...	You may be advised to reduce the dose of insulin that is active at the time you exercise. In general, adjusting insulin will depend on * the intensity of your exercise * the duration of your exercise * the type of insulin that is acting while you are exercising.

The table below provides some general guidelines for insulin adjustment during exercise:

Guidelines for insulin adjustment during Excercise

*Intensity of exercise**	*Duration of exercise*	*Per cent to Decrease Peaking Insulin***
Low to high	Less than 30 minutes	0 per cent
Low	30 - 60 minutes	5 per cent
Moderate	30 - 60 minutes	10 per cent
Moderate	60 or more minutes	20 per cent
High	30 - 60 minutes	20 per cent
High	60 or more minutes	30 per cent

* Low = not in target heart rate zone ** Irregular insulin - 2-4 hours after injecting
Moderate = low end of heart rate zone if NPH/Lente - 6 - 12 hours after injecting
High = high end of heart rate zone

You should take special precautions. Otherwise, the combination of insulin action and exercise may cause hypoglycemia. You should eat extra food before beginning the activity if you exercise when your insulin is peaking:

If you exercise during periods when your insulin is peaking...	If you will be exercising less than one hour, eat a snack containing 10 -15 grams of carbohydrate, such as a small piece of fresh fruit, 4 - 6 crackers, one slice of bread.
	If You will be exercising more than one hour, add 7 - 8 grams of protein to your snack, such as 1 ounce of low fat cheese, 1 ounce of poultry or lean meat, 1 tablespoon of peanut butter.
If you know in advance that you will be exercising when your insulin is peaking...	Reduce your dose of insulin which will peak at time by 10 -20 per cent, depending on the duration and intensity of the exercise.

Hypoglycemia

What are the signs of hypoglycemia (low blood glucose)?

If your treatment has been prescribed taking your diet and exercise in consideration, the chances for becoming hypoglycemic is not common, but you should be prepared and be able to recognize the signs and symptoms associated with a low blood glucose so that you can take preventive measures and not have a severe hypoglycemic reaction.

Classical signs and symptoms of hypoglycemia

Sympathoadrenal	Neuroglycopenic
Weakness	Headache
Sweating	Hypothermia
Tachycardia	Visual Disturbances
Palpitations	Mental dullness
Tremor	Confusion
Nervousness	Amnesia
Irritability	Seizures
Tingling	Coma
Huger	
Vomiting	

In case you experience any of these symptoms contact your doctor immediately.

Exercise.......Carry on!

Strategies for adhering to your exercise programme.

People with diabetes are often amazed at how well exercise can help them control their blood glucose. Even so, adhering to your exercise regimen can be difficult because it takes planning, time and discipline. Below are some strategies that you can use to help you maintain your exercise plans and continue to gain the benefits from your efforts:

- Choose exercise that you enjoy. It is easiest to avoid something that you don't like.
- Choose a variety of activities that you enjoy to prevent boredom.
- Set realistic goals for your exercise programme. If you set goals that are unrealistic for you, then you may become discouraged and quit.
- Keep your programme convenient to your lifestyle. Exercise is more rewarding if it doesn't interrupt the normal flow of your life.
- If you are self-conscious about exercising, find a group of people at a similar fitness level for companionship.
- Give yourself rewards for achieving your exercise goals.
- Exercise on a routine for achieving your exercise goals.

Aside from the physical benefits of exercise, it can give you a psychological boost, increasing your sense of well-being, your self-image and help you manage your stress better.

Energy requirements of common activities (Consumption of calories per minute).

Self-care Activities		**Recreational Activities**	
Rest, Supine	1.0	Painting, sitting	2.0
Sitting	1.2	Driving car	2.9
Standing	1.4	Skiing	9.9
Eating	1.4	Playing Squash	10.2
Conversation	1.4	Volleyball	3.5
Dressing, undressing	2.3	Bowling	4.4
Washing hand face	2.5	Cycling 5.5 mph	4.5
Walking 2.5 mph	3.6	Goly	5.0
Showering	4.2	Swimming, 20yd/min	5.0
Walking downstairs	5.2	Dancing	5.5
Walking upstairs	11.6	Gardening	5.6
		Tennis playing	7.1

Housework	
Hand sewing	1.4
Sweeping floor	1.7
Polishing furniture	2.4
Scrubbing standing	2.9
Floor	3.9
Making bed	3.9
Ironing standing	4.2
Mopping	4.2

Household Measures

1 Glass 240 ml	:	Height 4 1/2" Diameter on top 3" Diameter at bottom: 2"
1 Tablespoon	:	15g
1 Teaspoon	:	5g
1 Karchi	:	100g (Cooked weight)
1 cup 120 ml	:	Tea Cup height 2" Diameter 2"

Standard height and weights chart

Height		*Standard weight*			
		Men		*Women*	
		kg	*lbs*	*kg*	*lbs*
152.3 cm	(5'-0")	-	-	50.8-54.4	112-120
154.8 cm	(5'-1")	-	-	51.7-55.4	114-120
157.3 cm	(5'-2")	56.3-60.3	124-133	53.1-56.7	117-125
159.9 cm	(5'-3")	57.6-61.7	127-136	54.4-58.1	120-128
162.4 cm	(5'-4")	58.9-63.5	130-140	56.3-59.9	124-132
165.0 cm	(5'-5")	60.8-65.3	134-144	57.6-61.2	127-135
167.5 cm	(5'-6")	62.2-66.5	137-147	58.9-63.5	130-140
170.5 cm	(5'-7")	64.0-68.5	141-151	60.8-65.3	134-144
172.6 cm	(5'-8")	65.8-70.8	145-156	62.2-66.7	137-147
175.1 cm	(5'-9")	67.6-72.6	149-160	64.0-68.5	141-151
177.7 cm	(5'-10")	69.4-74.4	153-164	65.8-70.3	145-155
180.2 cm	(5'-11")	71.2-76.2	157-168	67.1-71.7	148-158
182.3 cm	(6'-0")	73.0-78.5	161-173	68.5-73.9	161-163
185.3 cm	(6'-1")	75.3-80.7	166-178	-	-
187.8 cm	(6'-2")	77.6-83.5	171-184	-	-
190.4 cm	(6'-3")	79.8-85.6	176-189	-	-

* *Courtesy*: Life Insurance Corporation of India.

Variety with Moderation

It is sometimes very monotonous to have a same diet routine for a diabetic. A variety can be included in diet plan by adding all the different kinds of foods by making the right choice or few changes. By this, you will not feel dissatisfied that you have left all the good things in the world and will also be motivated to stick to your diet regime as it will be full of variety.

South Indian Dishes

Most of the South Indian dishes can be taken by a diabetic. Idli, Uttapam, Sambhar, Dosa, all can be taken accordingly. Avoid vadas, rasam etc. which are fried. Avoid coconut chutney. Rava idli are preferred over rice idli. If making at home, add vegetable to it. Use non-stick for cooking uttapam, dosa etc. Dhokla and khandvi can be taken by a diabetic.

Chinese

In Chinese, always prefer steamed dishes instead of fried one. If having Chinese at a restaurant, ask the cook to use very less oil in fried rice or noodles. Avoid use of fried pieces of chicken in noodles or rice.

If preparing at home, add lot of vegetables to the noodles or rice. Don't add cornflour in chilly chicken or chill paneer. Same way don't add cornflour in soups. Instead chopped vegetables or wheat bran can be used to thicken it.

Avoid using butter or adding cream to the soup.

Fast Food Dishes

All the fast food dishes can be taken with few changes. In Pav Bhaji, don't add butter in Bhaji and Pav.

Pizzas can be taken occasionally with less or no cheese topping. Avoid fried toppings like fried chicken etc. Instead prefer vegetable topping. Try not to exceed more than 2 pcs. of pizza.

Burgers should be preferred with vegetable cutlet instead of potato cutlet in it. If preparing at home make cutlets in non-stick with very less oil. Avoid fried chicken filling and prefer grilled chicken pizza instead. While making the cutlets add wheat bran to the mixture of cutlet to increase the fibre content. Avoid adding cheese into it. Never order cheese burger. In a restaurant always prefer vegetable burger or grilled chicken burgers.

Sandwiches : Prefer having grilled sandwiches. Filling of boiled potato is preferred over vegetables with mayonnaise or cheese filling. Avoid using butter in the sandwich. While making at home, use brown bread. Even home-made Paneer can be added to the sandwich.

Mughlai Food

Always prefer grilled kababs instead of fried one. If in a restaurant, tell the cook not to add butter and cream to the dishes. Order normal tandoor chapatti instead of roomali roti or missi roti having desi ghee.

Italian/Mexican Food

Avoid sauces which are made from cream like mayonnaise etc. If preparing at home use skimmed milk curd instead as for example use curd instead of mayonnaise in Russian salad.

Sweets

Desserts can be taken by a diabetic by using sugar free instead of sugar. Custard, Apple Kheer, Rice Kheer, Fruit custard, Carrot Halwa etc. can be taken by preparing it in double toned milk.

Sugar, Jaggery, Honey should be avoided by the diabetics. Groundnut chikki, Gulabjamun, Kaju Burfi etc. should be avoided. Instead Rasgulla can be taken after squeezing it.

Recipes

Low Calorie Snacks, Salads and Desserts

For the controlled diabetes as well as individuals on low calorie diet with a sweet tooth, desserts may be permitted. The calories should be adjusted and free sugar should be avoided. Similarly, snacks and salads may be preferred occasionally as alternatives to routine.

Snacks

1. Broken Wheat Poha

No. of serving-1, size of serving-1 bowl
Broken wheat 10 gm
Moong sprouts 5 gm
Onion 10 gm
Carrot 15 gm
Fenugreek seeds 2 gm
Oil 2 gm

1. Pressure cook the broken wheat in double the volume of water till soft.
2. Wash and dice the carrots and chop onion finely.
3. Pressure cook the moong sprouts and carrots for two minutes or till soft.
4. Roast and grind the fenugreek seeds.
5. Saute the onion till light golden. Add the broken wheat, carrots and moong sprouts add salt and seasoning. Mix and cook for few minutes.
6. Garnish with coriander leaves and lemon.

Nutritive value/serving : Energy-80 K cal. Protein 3gm.

2. *Cabbage Roll*

No. of serving-1 ; size of serving-2 rolls
Cabbage leaf 40 gm
Sprouted black gram 10 gm
Oil 2 gm
Green chillies 5 gm
Curry leaves 5 gm
Mustard leaves - to taste
Coriander leaves - to taste
Lime juice - to taste

1. Sprout black gram and pressure cook it.
2. Blanch cabbage leaf.
3. Heat oil, add mustard, chillies, curry leaves and turmeric. Keep covered for 1/2 minute.
4. Add salt, lime juice, coriander and mix.
5. Add sprouted bengal gram to the mix.
6. Put the filling in the blanched cabbage.

Nutritive value/serving 73 K cal; Protein 2 gm.

3. *Dhokla*

No. of serving-1; size of serving-2 med. size.
Besan 15 gm
Curd 1-1/2 tsp
Green chillies 1
Ginger a small piece
Baking powder, pinch
Oil 2 gm
Coriander leaves 3 stalks
Peas 5 gm

1. Mix besan and curd, soak it overnight
2. Make a paste of ginger and green chillies and mix with the above batter.
3. Add salt, mix baking powder, a drop of oil and one tsp water and add to the mixture.

4. Grease a small plate and pour the batter into it and steam for 15-20 minutes.
5. Make coriander chutney.
6. Spread this chutney over one steamed pancake along with crushed boiled peas. Sandwich with one other pancake, spread remaining chutney on top and serve.

   Nutritive value/serving; 78 K cal. Protein 4 gm.

4. Egg Mouse

No. of serving 4
Gelatine 1-1/2 tsp.
Curry powder 1-1/2 tsp.
Salt and pepper to taste.
Cucumber, carrot, cabbage, tomatoes to garnish.
Finely chopped hard boiled eggs 4

1. Soak gelatine in 1 1/2 water, sprinkle gelatine over warm water, cup mix it.
2. Mix all other ingredients with gelatine.
3. Mould and refrigerate.
4. When set remove from mould and garnish with chopped and shredded cabbage, cucumber, tomato, etc.

   Nutritive value/serving 77 K cal; Protein 8 gm.

5. Fruit Tarts

No. of serving 1.
Size of serving 1.
Buck wheat flour 5 gm
Maize flour 5 gm
Soybean flour 5 gm
Curd (beaten) 10 gm
Egg (white) 15 gm
Apple 10 gm
Papaya 10 gm
Guava 10 gm

Moong sprout 5gm
Baking powder 1/4 tsp

1. Mix buck wheat flour, maize flour, soya flour and baking powder, sieve twice.
2. Fold egg white in flour
3. Add curd and water if required to make a softdough.
4. Roll out dough around 1/4 inch thick.
5. Cut with a biscuit cutter into rounds.
6. Lay in tray with tartlets making sure that they fit. Bake in moderate oven for 10 minutes.
7. Dice fruit and lemon juice and salt. Add sprouts. Mix, fill in tarts and serve.

Nutritive value/serving 82 K cal; Protein 6 gm.

6. *Low Calorie Idlis*

No. of serving 2, size of serving 2 med. Size
Urad dal 5 gm
Moong dal (whole) 5 gm
Ragi 20 gm
Cabbage 20 gm
Green Coriander
Curry leaves
Jeera to taste
Salt

1. Soak whole moong dal overnight. Leave it for sprouting.
2. Soak the ragi, urad dal overnight and grind them separately to a soft dough.
3. To the prepared dough, add salt and keep aside for fermentation.
4. Add shredded cabbage, chopped dhania and roasted jeera.
5. Smear the idli stand (plate) with little til oil and pour mixed dough.
6. Steam it.

Nutritive value/serving 88 K cal; Protein 3 gm.

7. Rainbow Sandwich

No. of serving 1; size of serving 2 sandwich
Besan 10 gm
Suji 5 gm
Moong sprouts 5 gm
Curd 5 gm
Tomatoes 40 gm
Mint chutney 1 tsp
Coriander leaves a few sprigs
Lemon juice 1 tsp
Mustard seeds 1/4 tsp.
Other spices
Red chilli powder
Jeera to taste
Haldi
Amchur

1. Roast suji. Then take roasted suji, besan, salt and other spices in bowl, add water. Mix well and make a thick batter.
2. Steam the batter for 10 minutes in a greased tin.
3. Let it cool for 15 minutes and then cut into 3 layers.
4. Now roast the mustard seeds, add coriander or curry leaves and mix with 2 tsp water, heat for a minute. Pour this mixture over 3 layers.
5. Blanch the tomatoes and make puree. Steam the sprouts.
6. Add the steamed sprouts to tomato puree and cook it to thicken. Add salt to taste.
7. On the bottom layer, spread mint chutney. Top it with 2nd layer. Spread tomato puree with sprouts. Top it with 3rd later. Serve garnished with coriander leaves and tomato slices.

   Nutritive value/serving 82 K cal; Protein 4 gm.

8. Soya Idlis

No. of serving 1; size of serving 2 idlis
Soybean flour 10gm
Suji 10 gm
Carrot 5 gm
Sprouts 5 gm
Mustard seeds 1/4 gm
Salt 1/2 tsp
Lemon juice 1/2 tsp
Curry leaves

1. Roast suji and soybean flour separately.
2. Make a batter adding water.
3. Roast mustard seeds till they crackle.
4. Add mustard seeds, salt and curry leaves to batter.
5. Put into idli cases and steam for 15 minutes.
6. Serve hot.

Nutritive value/serving, 80 K cal; Protein 3 gm.

9. Upma

No. of serving 1; size of serving 1 small bowl.
Suji 15 gm
Peas 20 gm
Tomato 10 gm
Onion 10 gm
Mustard seeds 1/2 tsp
Urad dal 1/2 tsp
Chana dal 1/2 tsp
Salt to taste
Refined oil 1/2 tsp

1. Heat oil and roast suji in it till slightly brownish.
2. In another skillet, heat some oil and saute mustard seeds, urad dal, chana dal then add chopped vegetable and simmer till slightly tender.
3. Boil water (1/2 cup).

4. Add suji to the sauted vegetable and add boiling water. Stir till done.
5. Serve hot.

Nutritive value/serving, 85 K cal. Protein 2 gm.

10. Vegetable Cheese Cake

No. of serving 2; size of serving 4 pieces
Flour 10 gm
Skimmed milk 150 gm
Cottage cheese 15 gm
Cauliflower
Peas 50 gm
Tomato
Carrot
Coriander leaves (a few sprigs)
Salt to taste
Black pepper as desired

1. Shell the peas. Chop finely all the vegetables and oil them. Blanch the tomatoes.
2. Grate the cheese.
3. Make white sauce. Add vegetable and grated cheese, salt and slowly stir the mixture till it thickens.
4. Grease the tin pour the mixture into it. Bake at 200°C for 15-20 minutes. Garnish with coriander leaves, tomato and serve.

Nutritive value/serving, 85 K cal; Protien 4 gm.

11. Vegetable Sausages

No. of serving ; size of serving 2
Cabbage 10 gm
Carrot 5gm
Chana dal 15 gm
Wheat flour 3 gm
Coriander powder 1/4 tsp.
Mango powder 1 pinch

Green chillies 2
Ginger 1 cm piece
Turmeric powder 1/8 tsp
Mustard seed 1 pinch
Lime half
Oil for frying

1. Soak the chana dal in water overnight and grind it to a paste along with the green chillies and ginger.
2. Grate the cabbage and carrot. Chop the coriander leaves finely.
3. Mix all ingredients from cabbage to turmeric powder a soft dough.
4. Divide the mixture into 2 portions. Put each portion in the firstfold and shape to form a sausage like roll.
5. Steam the rolls for about 10-15 minutes.
6. Heat oil. Add mustard seeds and let them burst. Add the steamed rolls and fry till light brown.
7. Serve hot garnished with coriander leaves and lime juice.

Nutritive value/serving, 80 K cal; Protein 4 gm.

Salads

1. Moong Raita

No. of serving 1; size of serving 1 medium bowl.
(Moong dal) Green gram (raw) 10 gm
Curd (skimmed) 100 gm
Cumin seeds
Pepper to taste
Salt
Coriander leaves few sprigs

1. Soak moong dal (whole) overnight in water, then tie it in a cloth to remove extra water. Alternatively, sprout the dal.
2. Cook the above in the pressure cooker for 2-3 minutes. Just steam it. Meanwhile beat the curd.

3. After cooking mix it in curd. Add seasoning and garnish with coriander leaves.

Nutritive value/serving, 80 K cal; Protein 6 gm.

2. *Corn Chaat*

No. of serving 1; size of serving 1 medium size bowl.
Fresh corn 50 gm
Onion 25 gm
Tomato 25 gm
Ginger
Green chillies
Coriander leaves
Salt to taste
Lemon juice

1. Steam fresh corn for 5 minutes.
2. Chop onion, tomato, ginger, chillies.
3. Mix all the ingredients together.
4. Serve chilled.

Nutritive value/serving, 70 K cal; Protein 4 gm.

3. *Fruit Sprout Chaat*

No. of serving 1; size of serving 1 bowl
Moong sprouts 10 gm
Orange 30 gm
Apple 25 gm
Guava 30 gm
Cucumber/Tomato 30 gm
Salt
Amchur
Black pepper to taste
Black salt
Roasted jeera

1. Sprout moong by soaking overnight and then hang it in wet muslin for a day or two, till sprouts appear.
2. Do not remove peel. Dice the fruits.

3. Add salt and spices to taste.

Nutritive value/serving, 85 K cal; Protein 3 gm.

4. *Garden Salad*

No. of serving 1; size of serving 1 cup
Mausami 1 medium
Papaya 30 gm
Apple 20gm
Cucumber 30 gm
Cottage cheese (skimmed) 10 gm
Salt and black pepper powder to taste

1. Scoop out the mausami pulp and extract the.juice
2. Dice papaya, apple and cucumber finely.
3. Crumble the cottage cheese.
4. Mix these into the juice.
5. Add salt and pepper powder.
6. Fill in the mausami cup and garnish.
7. Chill for an hour and serve cold.

Nutritive value/serving, 80 K cal; Protein 6 gm.

5. *Papaya Crunch*

No. of serving 2; size of serving 1 medium
Papaya 80 gm
Orange juice 10 ml
(skimmed) milk 20 ml
Cornflakes 10 gm
Egg white 1
Cinnamon powder 1/4 tsp
Oil 1/4 tsp

1. Dice peeled papaya and cook in water till tender.
2. Squeeze orange juice over it.
3. Boil milk and add a little cinnamon powder in it.

4. Beat egg white stiff and mix with papaya and milk.
5. Roll cornflakes in oil.
6. Place a layer of cornflakes on the base of a baking dish, pour mixture over it. Sprinkle rest of cinnamon powder and spread thin layer of cornflake over it.
7. Bake in a moderate oven for 20 minutes; serve.

Nutritive value/serving, 80 K cal; Protein 6 gm.

Low Calorie Desserts

In diabetes and in individuals on low calorie diet, fresh is the usual choice for dessert. Canned fruit packed in sugar syrup not to be used.

However, other desserts mentioned below, can be prepared and included in a diet with the substitution of different food exchanges mentioned along with the recipes.

Artificial sweetner available in the market can be used in place of sugar. It is estimated that one-fourth teaspoon of sweetex solution or 2 small tablets are equivalent to two teaspoons of sugar.

1. Lemon Gelatin

(Calories 25)
Unflavoured gelatin (1 tsp) 7 gm
Cold water 2 tsp
Lemon juice 1 tsp
Water 1/2 cup (120ml)
Aspartame (free Sugar) to taste

Heat cold water and add gelatin, dissolve and remove from stove. Add sweetex solution, lemon juice and 1/2 cup water. Chill and serve.

(make 1 serving)

2. *Fruit Jelly*

(Calories 65 or 1/2 and 1-1/2 fruit exchange)

Use 1 fruit orange or any fresh fruit or 1/2 cup orange juice in place of water in recipe for lemon gelatin chill and serve.

(make 1 serving)

3. *Fruity Ice*

(Calories 70)

Fresh orange or pineapple
Juice 120 ml
Lemon juice 1 tsp
Egg white 1
Water 1/2 cup (120 ml)

Combine fruit juice and water. Freeze. Stir mixture often while it is freeze. When almost hard, fold in stiffly beaten egg white. Cool and serve, (make 1 serving)

4. *Fresh Fruit Cup*

(Calories 40)
Water melon 300 gm
Or melon 300 gm
or orange/pear/apple/pineapple 100 gm

Scoop melon/water melon into balls with a scoop spoon and serve. (makes 1 serving)

5. *Baked Custard*

(Calories 160)
Milk 1/2 cup (120 ml)
Egg one
Salt few grains
Aspartame to taste
Vanilla essence

Beat one egg slightly, stir in milk, salt sweetex and vanilla. Pour into custard cups and set in hot water and bake at 350°F for about 45 minutes. (make 1 serving)

6. Carrot Halwa

(Calories 130)
Grated carrots 100 gm
Skimmed milk powder 20 ml
Or milk 1/2 cup 120 ml
Aspartame to taste

Cook grated carrots on slow heat, until soft. Add skimmed milk powder and mix well. Cook for 10 minutes. Remove from fire and add sweetex solution. Serve while hot (make 1 serving)

7. Kheer

(Calories 240)
Milk 200 ml
Rice/Suji 25gm
Elaichi/Kewra essence/Aspartame. These may be taken to taste.

Clean and pick rice/sieve suji. Boil milk with elaichi and add rice/suji. Cook till thick. Remove from stove and add kewra and sweetex (makes 1 saving)

8. Shree Khand

(Calories 80)
Soya granules 50gm
Wheat bran 10gm
Gur 50 gm
Ajwain to taste

Caramelize gur in dry hot pan, till it turns dark brown, thick paste. Add crushed soya granules and wheat bran into it, mix well on slow fire for about 10 minutes, till all granules get coated by caramelized gur. Take down from stove and put into a greased thali, compress down with hand. Cut into cubes. (makes 3 cubes)

10. Rasgulla

No. of serving 2; size of serving 2 rasgulla
(Skimmed milk) 400 ml
Cornflour 1 pinch
Citric acid 1/4 tsp
Sugar free tablets 5
(Aspartame)
Elaichi essence 2 drops
Water 2 cups

1. Heat milk. Allow it to cool.
2. Remove the cream.
3. Dissolve citric acid in 1 tsp water. Add slowly to the milk.
4. Tie the curdled milk in muslin cloth. Let the water drain.
5. Knead the curd and cornflour till smooth.
6. Make 4 balls of the mixture.
7. Boil water. Add the balls.
8. Boil for 15 minutes. Then cool.
9. Add essence, chill to serve.

Nutritive value/serving 80 K cal, Protein 3 gm.

11. Doughnut

No. of serving 5; size of serving 1 doughnut
Whole wheat flour 100gm
Milk powder 25gm
Gur (caramelized) 25gm
Baking powder 1/4 tsp
Oil for frying

1. Caramelize the gur.
2. Add little water and make a dough by adding baking powder and gur and fry adding hot water.
3. Leave it for 1/2 an hour.
4. Roll and shape it into a dough.

5. Deep fry in oil on a slow fire, till light brown in colour.

Nutritive value of each doughnut 80 K cal, Protein 2 gm.

12. *Baked Cheese Rounds*

No. of serving 1; size of serving 2 small rounds.

Cottage cheese (skimmed) 30 gm
Egg white 1/2
Apple 20 gm
Milk 10 ml
(Marie) biscuit crumbs 2.5 gm
Cardamom 1
Vanilla essence 102 drops
Aspartame (free sugar)

1. Heat milk to boil. Add lemon juice in a slow stream till milk curdles and clear water separates. Let it stand for 15 minutes and then strain it through a muslin cloth.
2. Meanwhile grease the paper cups and dust it with bread crumbs.
3. Chop the apply finely.
4. Mash the apple by using the milk.
5. Beat the egg while to stiff peak stage and fold into the above mixture. Now mix the apple into it.
6. Pour the above mixture into the tin and bake it at 200°C for 15-20 minutes.

Nutritive value/serving 88 K cal. Protein 2 gm.

13. *Black Forest Cake*

No. of serving 6; size of serving 12 pieces

6 separated eggs
100g wheat flour
25g cocoa
1/4 tsp salt sifted
1 tsp baking powder
1tsp vanilla essence.
For syrup

Sugar free (aspartame) tablets
1/2 cup water
To decorate:
100 gm (light, half and half) cream
15 sugar free tablets
Orange shreds 50gm
Chocolate
1 tsp cocoa
1 tsp milk
1 tsp flour
1 sugar free tablet
1/4 cup water

Whip egg yolks until light and creamy (mild). Mix in sifted ingredients and vanilla essence. Beat egg white with a pinch of baking powder and fold into yolk mixture. Pour into two 9" round tins brushed with melted butter. Bake for 30 minutes at 350°F in the oven. Cool, pour hot syrup over it, layer and cover with cream and spread chocolate and orange shreds over it. For chocolate, mix all the ingredients and cook for 2 minutes. Cool and freeze. Keep the cake in the fridge for at least 3 hours before serving.

14. Pumpkin Carrot Burfi

No. of serving 1; size of serving 2 burfi
Pumpkin 25 gm
Carrot 25 gm
Skimmed milk powder 20 gm
Melon seeds few for decoration.

1. Grate pumpkin and carrot.
2. Reconstitute the milk powder to milk.
3. Cook the mixture on slow flame until it gets thickened. Add pumpkin, carrot to it and mix well.
4. Grease the thali and set.
5. Decorate with melon seeds.

Nutritive value/serving 80 K cal, Protein 3 gm.

15. Tingling Rose Milk

No. of serving 1; size of serving 1 cup
Skimmed milk (cold) 150 ml
Rasna rose 2 tsp
Aspartame/saccharine drops 2 drops
Drinking soda 50 ml

1. Mix all the ingredients in the order listed.
2. Serve immdiately.

Nutritive value/serving 80 K cal, Protien 6 gm.

High Fibre (Bran) Preparations

1. Wheat Bran Biscuits (Salty)

Each biscuit contains 32 calories: 4 gm bran/biscuit
Wheat bran (choker) 100 gm
Refined wheat flour (maida) 100 gm
Ghee/oil 50 gm
Curd 50 gm
Ajwain and salt to taste.
Beat ghee till creamy.
Add curd and mix well.
Mix flour, bran, salt and ajwain.
Add prepared flour to the curd mixture and make dough.
Keep it covered for 4-5 hours.
Roll out and cut into required shapes.
Bake at 350°F for 25-30 minutes or until done.
Make 25 biscuits.

2. Wheat Bran Biscuits (Sweet)

Each biscuit contains 40 calories; 4 gm bran/biscuit
Wheat brant (choker) 100 gm
Refined wheat flour (maida) 100 gm
Ghee/oil 50 gm
Gur 50 gm (caramelized)

beat ghee till creamy.
Add flour bran, crushed caramelized gur and make dough.
Keep it for 4-5 hours.
Roll out and cut into required shapes.
Bake at 350°F for 25-30 minutes or until done.
Make 25 biscuits.

3. *Bran Muffins*

Each muffin contains 35 calories; 8 gm bran/muffin
Wheat bran 100 gm
Refined wheat flour (maida) 100 gm
Curd/paneer 50 gm
Gur 50 gm (caramelized)
Egg 1
Baking powder 1/4 tap
Milk to make batter

Make a mixture of crushed gur with curd/paneer.
Mix baking powder into the refined flour.
Mix refined flour and bran into the curd mixture.
Add slightly beaten egg.
Pour into individual cups.
Bake at 350°F (for 30-35 minutes).
Make 12 muffins.

4. *Soya Bran Upma*

80 calories/serving.
Nutrinugget/Nutrella granules 50 gm
(Soybean product)
Bran 50 gm
Cooking oil 5 gm (1 tsp)
Curry patta a few
Mustard seeds (Rye) one pinch
Haldi
Hing

Salt to taste
Adrak (Ginger)
Chopped green chillies

Roast bran separately in dry frying pan/Karahi.

Moisten soya granules in a little water.

Add oil in a pan. Beat and add hing, mustard seeds, haldi, curry patta, green chillies and ginger.

Add roasted bran and soya granules into the above oil. Add salt mix well and cook for 10 minutes on slow fire.

Serve with fresh lemon.

Makes three servings.

5. *Bran Chapati*

Each chapati contains 40 calories; 5 gm bran/chapati.
Wheat flour (atta) 50 gm
Bran 20 gm

Make dough of both, together with water. Leave for sometime, about half an hour.

Roll into chapatis and cook.

Make four chapatis.

6. *Bran Bread*

Each slice contains 35 calories; 3.5 gm bran/slice
Bran 100 gm
Refined wheat flour (maida)
Cooking oil and ghee 25 gm
Yeast 8-10 gm
Water 100 gm

Dissolve yeast in warm water.

Mix all ingredients with yeast, water and make dough.

Keep dough in tin for 1-2 hours.

Bake at 350°F (until done).

Make one loaf with 24 slices.

7. Dahi Vada

Calories 125/ serving of two vadas
Urad dhuli dal 25 gm
Curd 250 gm
Bran 100 gm
Salt to taste
Roasted jeera (cumin) 1 tsp
Ginger small piece.
Black pepper to taste
Soak dal overnight.

Grind dal, bran and ginger together to thick batter consistency.

Make balls and fry them.

Beat curd, add roasted jeera powder and salt and pepper to taste.

Soke vadas in water, squeeze and soak them in the curd.

Make six servings two vadas each serving.

8. Bran Tikka

35 calories; 8 gm bran/tikka
Chana dal 25 gm
Bran 100 gm
Ginger (adrak) 1 small piece
Garlic (lassun) 8-10 cloves
Cardamon (ilaichi) 2-3 cloves
Cumin seeds (jeera) few seeds
Salt to taste

Cook chana dal till slightly soft.
Grind dal and above ingredients to a fine paste.
Mix bran with a little water and add to the above mixture. Mix well.
Make small balls with hand, flatten slightly and deep fry.
Serve with tomato ketchup/pudina or dhania chutney.
Make 12 tikkas.

Diet Charts

Diet chart for diabetic children

(24 Hours intake)

Meal	Menu	Weight/Measure
Early morning	-Milk	-1 cup
Breakfast	-Cereal product	-2 in no. (60 gms raw)
	-Paneer / Egg	-30 gms/2 in no.
	-Butter	-3/4 tea spoon
Mid-day	-Fruit	-100
Lunch Break	-Chapati	-2 in no. (60 gms raw)
	-Vegetable	-1 katori
Lunch	-Salad	-1plate
	-Chapati / Rice	-3 in no.
	-Vegetable	-1 katori
	-Dal	-1 katori
	-Curd or Paneer	-200 gms or 30 gms
Evening	-Milk	-250 ml
	-Snack	-equiv. to 2 chapati
	-Fruit	-100 gms
Dinner	-Salad / Soup	-1 plate/1 bowl
	-Chapati	-3 in no.
	-Vegetable	-1 katori
	-Dal	-1 katori
	-Curd or non-veg	-200 gms or 60 gms

1800 Kcal (40 gms protein)
(24 Hours intake)

Meal	Menu	Weight/Measure
Early morning	-Tea	-1 cup
	-Marrie Biscuit	-4-5 in no.
Breakfast	- Chapati or dalia	-2 in no. or 50 gms raw
	Contents	**Grams** or sabutdana
	-Potato	-50 gms
	-Milk	-1 cup (200ml)
	Egg (opt.)	1 white
Mid-day	-Fruit	-200 gms
	-Upma or murmura	1 Katori (60 gms)
Lunch	-Chapati	-2-3 in no.
	-Vegetable	-1 katori
	-Potato	-50 gms
	-Curd	-100 gms
Evening	-Tea	-1 cup (25 ml milk)
	-Paneer sandwich	-2 breads + paneer 25 gms
	Or idli	-2 in no.
Dinner	-Chapati	-2 in no.
	-Rice	-1 katori
	-Vegetable	-1 katori
	-Curd or fish or	-100 gms
	Chicken	or 25 gms
Permitted oil amts.	Any refined oil	4 tea spoons (20ml)

1200 Kcal diet chart
(24 Hours intake)

Meal	Menu	Weight/Measure
Early morning	-Tea	-1 cup (30 ml.)
	-Marie Biscuit	-2 in nos.
Breakfast	-Chapati	-1 in no. (25 gms raw)
	-Vegetable	-1 katori (free veg.)
	-Milk/Lassi	-1 cup/1 glass
Mid-day	-Fruit	-100 gms
	-Snack	equiv. to 1 chapati
Lunch	-Salad	1 plate
	-Chapati/Rice	-2 in no. (50 gms raw)
	-Vegetable	-1 katori
	-Dal or	-1 katori (25 gms) or
	Curd	-1/2 katori (100 gms)
Evening	-Tea	-1 cup (milk 30 ml)
	-Snack	equiv. to 1 chapati
Dinner	-Salad/Soup	1 plate
	-Chapati	-2 in no. (50 gms raw)
	-Vegetable	-1 katori
	-Dal or non-veg or	-1 katori or 50 gms or
	Curd	100 gms
Permitted oil amts.	Any refined oil	2 tea spoons

1400 Kcal diet chart
(24 Hours intake)

Meal	Menu	Weight/Measure
Early Morning	-Tea	-1 cup (milk 30 ml.)
	-Marie Biscuit	-2 in nos.
Breakfast	-Chapati	-2 in no. (50 gms raw)
	-Vegetable	-1 katori (free veg.)
	-Milk/Curd	-1 cup/100 gms (1/2 katori)
	-Egg/Paneer (opt.)	-1 in no./30 gms
Mid-day	-Fruit	-100 gms
	-Lemon water	-1 glass
Lunch	-Salad	1 plate
	-Chapati /Rice	-2 in no. (50 gms raw)
	-Vegetable	-1 katori
	-Dal	-3/4 katori (25 gms)
	-Curd	-1/2 katori (100gms)
Evening	-Tea	-1 cup
	-Snack	equiv. to 1 chapati
Dinner	-Salad/Soup	1 plate/1 bowl
	-Chapati	-2 in no. (50 gms raw)
	-Vegetable	-1 katori
	-Dal or non-veg	-1 katori or 60 gms
Permitted oil amts.	Any refined oil	2 tea spoons (10 ml)

1500 Kcal (30 gms protein)
(24 Hours intake)

Meal	Menu	Weight/Measure
Early Morning	-Tea	-1 cup (milk 25 ml.)
	-Marie Biscuit	-4-5 in no.
Breakfast	-Chapati or dalia or sabutdana	-2 in no. or 50 gms raw
	-Potato	-50 gms
	-Milk	-1 cup (200 ml)
	-Egg (opt.)	-1 white
Mid-day	-Fruit	-200 gms
	-Murmura or Paneer sandwich (opt.)	30 gms/ 1bread slice/ paneer - 25 gms
Evening	-Tea	-1 cup (30 ml milk)
	-Veg. sandwich or Marie Biscuits	-1 bread/4 in no.
Dinner	-Salad	-1 plate (no salt)
	-Chapati	-2 in nos.
	-Vegetable	-1 katori
	Curd	-100 gms
Permitted oil amts.	Any refined oil	4 tea spoons (20 ml)

1600 Kcal diet chart
(24 Hours intake)

Meal	Menu	Weight/Measure
Early Morning	-Tea	-1 cup (milk 30 ml.)
	-Marie Biscuit	-4 in no.
Breakfast	-Chapati	-2 in no. (50 gms raw)
	-Vegetable	-1 katori
	-Milk/Curd	-1 cup/200 gms
Mid-day	-Fruit or	-200 gms or
	Snack	-equiv. to 1 chapati
Lunch	-Salad	1 plate
	-Chapati	-2 in no. (50 gms)
	-Vegetable	-1 katori
	-Dal	-3/4 katori (25 gms)
	-Curd	-1 katori (200gms)
Evening	-Tea	-1 cup (30 ml milk)
	-Snack	equiv. to 1 chapati
Dinner	-Salad/Soup	-1 plate/1 bowl
	-Chapati	-2 in no. (50 gms raw)
	-Vegetable	-1 katori
	-Dal or non-veg or	-3/4 katori or 60 gms or
	Paneer	30 gms
Bed time	-Milk	-1 cup (250 ml)
Permitted oil amts.	Any refined oil	3 tea spoons (15 ml)

1800 Kcal diet chart
(24 Hours intake)

Meal	Menu	Weight/Measure
Early Morning	-Tea	-1 cup (milk - 30 ml.)
	Marie Biscuit	-4 in nos.
Breakfast	-Chapati	-2 in nos. (50 gms raw)
	-Vegetable	-1 katori
	-Milk/Curd	-1 cup/200 gms
	-Egg/Paneer	-2 in no. 30 gms
Mid-day	-Fruit	-200 gms
	-Snack	-equiv. to 1 chapati
Lunch	-Salad	-1 plate
	-Chapati	-2 in no. (50 gms raw)
	-Vegetable	-1 katori
	-Dal	-3/4 katori (25 gms)
	-Curd	-3/4 katori (150 gms)
Evening	-Tea	-1 cup
	-Snack	equiv. to 1 chapati
Dinner	-Salad/Soup	1 plate/1 bowl
	-Chapati	-3 in no. (75 gms raw)
	-Vegetable	-1 katori
	-Dal or non-veg	-3/4 katori/60 gms
	-Curd	-1/2 katori (100 gms)
Bed time	-Milk	-1 cup (250 ml)
Permitted oil amts.	Any refined oil	3 tea spoons (15 ml)

2000 Kcal diet chart
(24 Hours intake)

Meal	Menu	Weight/Measure
Early Morning	-Tea	-1cup (milk 30 ml.)
	-Marie Biscuit	-4 in nos.
Breakfast	-Chapati	-2 chapati (50 gms raw)
	-Vegetable	-1 katori
	-Milk/Curd	-1 cup/200 gms
	-Egg/Paneer	-2 whites/30 gms
Mid-day	-Fruit	-200 gms
	-Snack	-equiv. to 1 chapati
Lunch	-Salad	-1 plate
	-Chapati/Rice	-3 chapati (75 gms raw)
	-Vegetable	-1 katori
	-Dal	-3/4 katori (25 gms)
	-Curd	-3/4 katori (125 gms)
Evening	-Tea	-1 cup (milk 30 ml)
	-Snack	equiv. to 1 chapati
Dinner	-Salad/Soup	-1 plate/1 bowl
	-Chapati	-3 chapati (75 gms raw)
	-Vegetable	-1 katori
	-Dal or non-veg	-3/4 katori (25 gms)/60 gms
	-Curd	-3/4 katori (150 gms)
Bed time	-Milk	-1 cup (250 ml)
Permitted oil amts.	Any refined oil	3 tea spoons (15 ml)

Special Situations Requiring Dietary Modifications

1. Fasting

Can a diabetic fast? This would depend on whether one is a Type I insulin dependent diabetic on insulin therapy, or Type II non-insulin dependent diabetic on oral hypoglycaemic agents. The absence of insulin and food in IDDM may lead to coma in Type I Diabetic.

Fasting is thus only advised in the non-insulin dependent Type II diabetics, as metabolic adjustments in such individuals can be tolerated and this helps in reduction of weight.

Periodic fasting undertaken at regular intervals is well tolerated in NIDDM and if the person adjusts to the regime, weight reduction should be the objective of such a practice. By complete fasting an adult can lose approximately 0.4 kg in one day. An overweight diabetic is encouraged to fast once a week, when the patient is not on insulin or any other oral medication.

2. Sick days

In the case of any sickness, a diabetic on insulin or oral drugs must consult a doctor even though the illness might not seem serious. The physician will advise the dose of the anti-diabetic agent and modify the diet accordingly. Till thus advised, one should keep taking fluids or items like thin soup, buttermilk, tea or fresh lime.

In the event of fever or other illness, the diabetic diet should be modified by changing the consistency and texture of foods.

During sickness, the diabetic has to be very careful that acetone does not appear in the urine as it can lead to coma.

- Continue the daily dose of insulin.
- Those on oral drugs may discontinue tablets (especially if on biguanide); it may be safer to go back to an equivalent dose of insulin; consult your treating physician.
- It will be better to have somebody at home to take care of the diabetic and be easily accessible for any assistance.
- If in doubt, inform/consult your doctor at the earliest.
- Take plenty of fluids (fresh lime with salt, clear soups, buttermilk and an added intake of salt should be encouraged).
- If there is no nausea/vomiting, light meals may be taken (half boiled/poached egg, toast, khichri, curd and fruits are acceptable).

3. Travelling

The timing of meals may have to be adjusted. This would mean adjustment in the schedule of insulin or oral drugs to what is being taken as food. One should carry nutritious snacks while travelling, as they may be of additional help, in timing a major meal. This would also safeguard one from eating wayside foods, the chances of infection, or inaccessibility in case one is unwarily delayed on way due to the late schedule of the transport one is travelling. Some biscuits, a tin of cheese or some home-made snacks are easy item to carry and can replace a cooked meal. Something like sweet (chocolate, candy) should also be carried as it helps in the event of early symptoms of hypoglycaemia. It would be beneficial to always carry an identification card which declares that one is a diabetic and is on a particular medication for this purpose. This would facilitate diagnosis and timely management in case of an emergency.

4. At Parties/Eating Out

The most important fact is to have confidence and be discreet in calculating the calories. One should not make onself or one's host conscious of being a diabetic. Self-restraint is a great virtue. Select foods that are plainly cooked without too much of oil and sugar. Avoid cereals, rich gravies and meats with fats. For example, in chicken curry, eat just the chicken pieces and leave the curry aside or in dahi vada, eat only the dahi and leave vada alone. Salads add to the bulk of food and at the same time make the plate look full. Some fresh fruits can be opted for as dessert. At a birthday party, a diabetic child may share the cake, but manage with a smaller helping (50% of what other take), go in for fruit chat or chana chat or plain biscuits. Estimate the extra calories and adjust these in the next meal or go for a brisk and long walk to use them up. If one can learn to eat slowly, one can easily avoid second or third helpings.

The purpose of a diet for a diabetic is not to deny him food but rather to enable him to select the right items in appropriate amounts. A strict diabetic programme is the mainstay of any diabetic treatment. The care exercised in the direction is well rewarded. Maximum emphasis is on the calorie count.

Calories Values

Breakfast Food

Foodstuff	Calories	Fat Saturated (gm)	Total (gm)	Chole-sterol (mg)
Bacon Fried 1 slice (25gms)	95	2.8	9.0	3.0
Bread, White 2 Slice (40 gms)	98	-	0.3	-
Bun 1 big (60 gms)	170	-	0.4	-
Cheese Toast 2 Slice (70 gms)	220	8.0	13.1	19.5
Corn Flakes 1 cup without milk & sugar	95	-	Traces	-
Dosa-Masala/Mysore With butter (200gms)	400	9.0	25.0	42.0
Dosa, plain (50 gms)	200	7.0	10.0	-
Egg, white 1 white (17gms)	15 -	-	-	
Egg whole (50 gms)	87	1.7	6.6	248.0
Egg, Yolk 1 yolk (33gms)	62	1.7	6.6	248.0
Egg, Boiled (50 gms)	87	1.7	6.6	248.0
Egg (fried/omelette/scrambled)				
(a) suing 1 tbsp. (15gm) butter/ghee	200	16.1	18.7	290.0
(b) using 1 tbsp. Oil	225	11.2	21.6	248.0
Finger Chips 1 serving	465	21.0	30.2	-

Foodstuff	Calories	Fat Saturated (gm)	Total (gm)	Cholesterol (mg)
Fruit Bread 1 slice (20gms)	60	0.1	1.0	-
Ham, Roasted 1 slice (gms)	245	10.4	25.0	25.0
Idli with sambar (60gms)	250	1.0	5.0	-
Luncheon Meat 1 slice (20gms)	65	1.7	5.0	3.0
Milk bread 1 slice (20gms)	55	0.1	5.0	0.2
Milk, skimmed 1 cup (200ml)	74	-	0.2	0.4
Milk, whole 1 cup (200ml)	150	4.9	8.1	22.0
Phoe (Potato)	240	3.5	8.0	-
Parotha, Plain (50gms)	250	7.0	12.5	28.0
Parotha, stuffed (70gms)	300	7.0	12.5	28.0
Sausages, Cooked (25gms)	85	1.6	7.0	25.0
Salami 1 slice (10gms)	45	3.1	7.0	-
Tomato Omelette (60gms)	250	7.0	12.0	-
Uttappam, Onion (75gms)	275	7.0	10.8	-
Upma 1 plate (150gms)	235	3.5	8.0	-
Snacks 'N' Savouries				
Belpuri 1 plate (150gms)	185	3.5	5.5	-
Biscuits, slated (10gms)	53	0.3	3.2	-

Foodstuff	Calories	Fat Saturated (gm)	Total (gm)	Cholesterol (mg)
Biscuits, Sweet (10gms)	45	0.1	1.3	-
Cutlets, Mutton (200gms)	480	18.5	28.5	95.0
Cutlets, Vegetable (200gms)	450	17.5	25.0	-
Dahi Vada (60gms)	250	10.5	19.5	-
Farsan/Chewada 1 plate (100gms)	230	10.5	15.0	-
Kachoris (150gms)	400	14.0	20.0	-
Patties (200gms)	300	7.0	10.0	-
Paneer pakoda (50gms)	275	15.2	22.0	20.0
Pizza (Meat) 1 small (225gms)	400	14.5	20.0	75.0
Pizza (Vegetable, cheese) 1 small (200gms)	325	11.7	15.0	32.5
Potato Wadas (150gms)	470	14.0	20.0	-
Puri Bhaji 1 plate (250gms)	685	27.0	42.0	-
Ragada patties 1 plate (250gms)	450	7.0	13.0	-
Samosa (150gms)	500	14.0	20.0	-
Sev Puri 1 plate (200gms)	225	10.5	15.0	-
Bhajias, Onion 1 plate (150gms)	395	17.5	27.6	-
Cauliflower Pakoras 1 plate (150gms)	410	17.5	27.9	-
Almonds (100gms)	655	4.2	58.9	-

Foodstuff	Calories	Fat Saturated (gm)	Total (gm)	Cholesterol (mg)
Cashewnuts (100gms)	596	9.3	46.9	-
Pistachios (100gms)	680	7.8	57.8	-
Walnuts (100gms)	687	6.6	64.5	-
Meals				
a. Soups				
Chicken Soup 1cup	185	6.8	12.5	87.0
Chicken Vegetable soup 1 cup	162	4.4	8.7	73.0
Corn Soup (Sweet) 1 cup	120	1.7	7.0	248.0
Dal Soup 1 cup	137	2.2	4.2	14.0
Green Peas Soup 1 cup	176	2.2	5.5	14.0
Spinach Soup 1 cup	50	2.2	4.4	14.0
Tomato Soup 1 cup	87	2.2	4.2	14.0
Each cup equivalent to 200ml				
b. Salads				
Russian Salad 1 serving (100gm)	545	18.1	50.0	289
Sprouted Pulse Salad 1 serving (100gm)	225	3.5	5.7	-
c. Vegetable				
Brinjal Bhartah 1 serving (150gm)	150	7.0	10.5	-
Chana masala 1 serving (200gm)	240	7.0	10.0	-
Chana Dal 1 bow/1 cup (150gms)	270	7.0	17.8	-

Foodstuff	Calories	Fat Saturated (gm)	Total (gm)	Chole-sterol (mg)
Dum Aloo 1 serving (150gm)	254	10.8	15.7	1.6
Macaroini and Tomato (butter) 1 serving (100gm)	396	15.4	27.3	70
Mixed Vegetables- Carrots Peas, Cauliflower, Beans etc. 1 serving (150gm)	175	7.0	10.5	-
Palak Paneer 1 serving (150gm)	180	11.0	13.0	20.0
Potato and peas 1 serving (150gm)	235	7.0	10.0	-
Paneer Tikka 1 serving (150gm)	285	16.4	25.0	42.3
Potato Vegetable 1 serving (150gm)	165	7.0	11.2	-
MEALS				
Dalbhaji (Spinach and Bengal Gram Dal) 1 serving (150gm)	125	3.5	7.0	-
Stuffed Bhindi 1 serving (150gm)	200	3.5	7.0	-
Stuffed capsicum 1 serving (150gm)	120	3.5	6.2	-
Stuffed Karela 1 serving (150gm)	275	17.5	28.5	-
Usal 1 serving (150gm)	160	3.5	5.5	-
Vegetables, Leafy 1 serving (150gm)	100	3.5	5.5	-
Vegetables, Baked 1 serving (150gm)	395	6.7	22.5	5.3
d. Cereals				
Bhakri (Jowar, Bajra, Ragi) 1 med. (90gms)	300	-	1.5	-

Foodstuff	Calories	Fat Saturated (gm)	Total (gm)	Chole-sterol (mg)
Biryani Mutton 1 med. Bowl (150gms)	255	11.5	16.5	-
Chapati 1 med. (30 gms)	100	-	0.5	-
Chapati with ghee 1 tsp 1 med. (30 gms)	150	2.3	5.5	-
Fired Rice 1 med. Bowl (150 gms)	20	5.2	7.5	-
Khichri 1 serving (150 gms)	190	3.5	10.0	-
Naan 1 no. (20gms)	225	2.1	3.4	-
Puris 1 no. (20 gms)	105	4.2	6.2	-
Pulao, Vegetable 1 med. Bowl (100gms)	170	3.5	5.0	-
Rice cooked 1 med. Bowl (100gms)	100	-	-	-
Khadi 1 bowl/cup (200ml)	150	7.5	11.0	2.7
Kofta Curry 1 serving (200ml)	225	10.0	15.0	-
Lauki Dal 1 bowl/cup (200ml)	150	7.0	11.5	-
Rajma Curry 1 bowl/cup (200ml)	290	7.0	10.7	-
Prawn Pulao 1 serving	510	7.3	32.5	150
Egg Fried Rice 1 serving	280	1.7	16.7	248
NON-VEGETARIAN				
Beef Curry 1 serving	185	8.0	11.0	100
Chicken Butter 1 serving	305	11.4	21.0	160

Foodstuff	Calories	Fat Saturated (gm)	Total (gm)	Chole-sterol (mg)
Chicken Curry 1 serving	175	7.1	10.4	70
Chicken Chilli 1 serving	255	10.5	16.0	90
Chicken Fried in Butter 1 serving	440	15.0	25.5	217
Chicken Paella 1 serving	325	10.5	15.8	45
Chicken Patties 2 pieces	325	14.0	20.4	45
Chopsuey 1 serving	150	7.3	11.4	18
Egg Curry 1 serving	235	12.4	21.5	248
Elaichi Mutton 1 serving	215	1.5	13.6	70
Fish Baked 1 serving	395	8.7	32.3	107
Fish Curry 1 serving	35	3.5	7.0	50
Fish & Chips 1 serving	850	35.2	52.8	130
Fish in Curds (Hilsa) 1 serving	505	14.5	40.5	82
Fish Fried 1 piece (50 gms)	220	10.5	17.5	50
Kheema Mutter 1 serving	240	8.5	13.6	70
Mutton Curry 1 serving	185	8.0	12.7	95
Mutton Vindaloo 1 serving	334	18.5	28.6	70
Nargisi Kabab 2 pieces	360	17.0	29.3	301
Pork Curry 1 serving	185	8.3	13.5	80

Foodstuff	Calories	Fat Saturated (gm)	Total (gm)	Chole-sterol (mg)
Pork Sorpote (Goan) 1 serving	321	15.4	25.1	165
Prawns Fried 1 serving	273	14.1	21.0	150
Prawn malaya Curry 1 serving	415	28.0	32.4	150
Stewed Mutton 1 serving	145	4.5	7.5	95
Stuffed Mutton Malai Kofta 1 serving	600	27.0	50.0	215
Sweet and Sour Mutton 1 serving	285	10.5	20.5	176

Each serving equivalent to 150 gms unless indicated otherwise

Foodstuff	Calories	Fat Saturated (gm)	Total (gm)	Chole-sterol (mg)
ORGAN MEAT				
Brain (100gms)	107	2.4	8.5	235
Heart Beef, Goat (100gms)	115	1.5	5.0	256
Kidney Goat (100gms)	120	4.2	11.0	700
Liver				
Beef (100gms)	110	2.6	5.3	406
Goat (100gms)	107	2.6	5.3	406
Lamb (100gms)	110	2.8	6.8	510
Pork (100gms)	110	2.9	5.5	420
SEA FOOD				
Crabs Cooked (75gms raw)	155	-	10.5	70
Prawns, Cooked (75gms raw)	155	-	10.5	70
Lobsters (75gms raw)	165	-	12.0	70

Foodstuff	Calories	Fat Saturated (gm)	Total (gm)	Chole-sterol (mg)
SWEETS AND DESSERTS				
Amriti (50gms)	295	10.5	16.0	-
Basundi	270	6.0	12.0	27.5
1 serving (150gms)				
Besan Ladoo (50gms)	205	5.5	8.5	-
Bundi Ladoo (50gms)	210	5.2	8.5	-
Cake, Iced	190	4.8	8.0	50.0
1 slice (40gms)				
Custard, Plain	220	5.0	8.2	22.0
1 serving (200gms)				
Custard with Jelly	230	5.0	8.2	22.0
1 serving (225gms)				
Fruit Salad	250	5.0	8.2	22.0
1 serving (225gms)				
Gulab Jamun (60gms)	282	13.0	20.2	12.5
Halwa, Vegetable	225	7.0	13.7	42.0
(carrot, pumpkin, gourd)				
1 serving (200gms)				
Ice-Cream (Small)	215	6.7	10.8	45.0
1 cup (100gms)				
Jalebi (40gms)	280	10.5	16.0	-
Kheer, Rice	240	3.6	8.0	22.0
1 avg. serving (200gms)				
Kheer, Vermicelli	240	3.6	8.5	22.0
1 serving (200gms)				
Modak, Fried (40gms)	250	11.0	19.5	-
Pudding, Bread	300	7.0	15.3	5.0
1 serving (150gms)				
Pudding, Milk	280	7.0	14.8	58.0
1 serving (150gms)				
Puran Poli (60gms)	315	14.0	26.0	-
Rasgulla (40gms)	180	2.4	4.2	7.0
Rewal Ladoo (50gms)	205	5.2	8.5	-
Rasmalai, 2 Rasgullas	370	9.6	12.5	29.0
1 serving (150gms)				